THE DIABETIC COOKBOOK

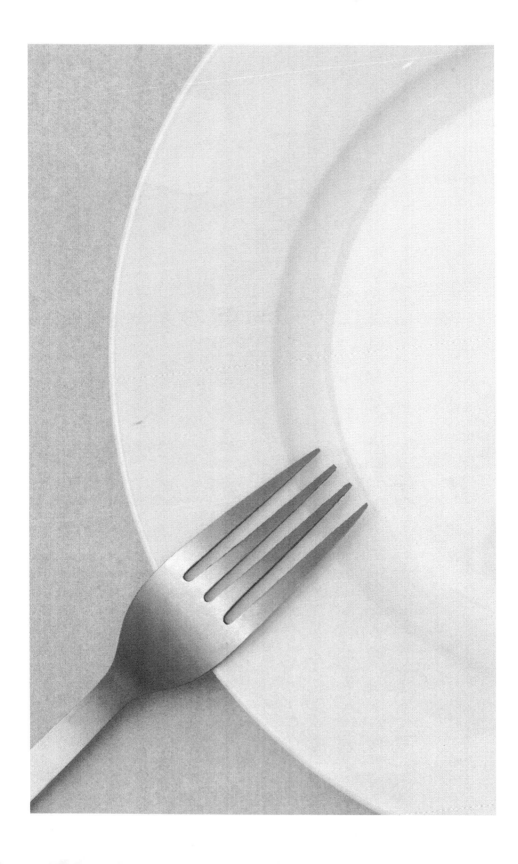

THE
Diabetic
Cookbook

Easy, Healthy, and **Delicious**
Recipes for a **Diabetes Diet**

SHASTA PRESS

Contents

CHAPTER THREE

Small Bites   34

CHAPTER FOUR

Snacks and Dips   52

CHAPTER EIGHT

Vegetable Side Dishes   130

CHAPTER NINE

Vegetarian Entrées   146

CHAPTER TEN

Pastas   168

CHAPTER ELEVEN

Seafood and Poultry Dishes   190

Introduction

They Don't Call It Comfort Food for Nothing

We all have special memories of our childhood, and a good number of them center around food. Whether it was a special celebration, holiday, Sunday dinner, Saturday breakfast, or even just ordinary weekday meal, chances are your kitchen was the heart of your home. Home and hearth; family and friends gathered around the table sharing a meal or maybe just dessert; the familiar smells of oatmeal chocolate-chip cookies, lemonade, meat loaf, baked beans, breads, and pies wafting from the kitchen make for powerful memories. Food can be comforting to the mind as well as the body, and sharing delicious food made from scratch is the ultimate expression of love. You can taste the care that went into it. When food is made with love, it is simply better. It's interesting how new cuisines come into vogue, but the comforting and familiar dishes made in the warm, fragrant kitchens of our childhood are the ones we crave.

These comfort foods aren't fancy. But for most of us, the ordinary dinner of tuna casserole or picnic with savory pork and beans is what tasted the best, and often these recipes are what have been passed down through the generations. Eating Grandma's baked beans or Mom's vegetable soup makes us feel good. It's the ordinary, everyday home-cooked foods that taste the best and still bring us the most comfort.

As with everything, food has evolved. Those traditional and cozy dishes typically are high in calories, sugar, and fat. But with our knowledge of modern healthful cooking techniques and fresh ingredients, there is no reason we can't still enjoy our favorite comfort foods. This book reintroduces you to the familiar foods you love to eat, but this time they're prepared so they can be enjoyed by everyone, including those with diabetes, and they taste as good as you remember. No longer is there any need to cook "special" diabetic meals when everyone sits down together to share the same meal and continue to make new memories around the table.

This book will be especially helpful to those who are newly diagnosed with diabetes. Knowing how to eat healthfully and manage portion size goes a long way toward making it easier to live with this disease. When everyone can eat the same meal and not feel deprived, people with diabetes, friends, and family do not need to give up their favorite foods, and the family cook doesn't have to do double duty in the kitchen. Cooking and eating can still be one of life's great pleasures, shared with loved ones of all ages.

The recipes in this book are simple to follow: cheeseburgers, French fries, spaghetti, potpie, vanilla ice cream, chocolate-chip cookies, macaroni and cheese, apple pie, mashed potatoes, meat loaf—the list includes 150 favorite American classics. Recipes ranging from regional American classics to ethnic favorites are revisited and made diabetes-friendly, and newer favorites like fajitas and curry noodle soup are given a fresh twist. And let's not forget the old standbys: tuna, green bean, sweet potato, and broccoli casseroles are also given a makeover, as are all of the mayonnaise-based salads that are so popular at picnics, like macaroni salad, potato salad, and coleslaw.

If you're wondering how these recipes can be more nutritious but also be more flavorful and still taste familiar, the answer is in using high-quality low-fat cheeses, small amounts of real butter, kosher salt, fresh herbs, spices, good-quality olive oil, the ripest produce, and the best poultry, seafood, and meats. When the ingredients are of good quality and prepared from scratch, food tastes good. It's that simple. Be a selective shopper, and use the recommended ingredients for these recipes, which can be easily found. You'll end up with flavor-rich dishes that your family and friends will love.

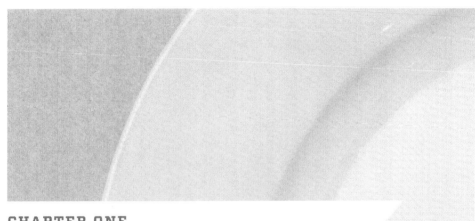

CHAPTER ONE

Smart Food Choices

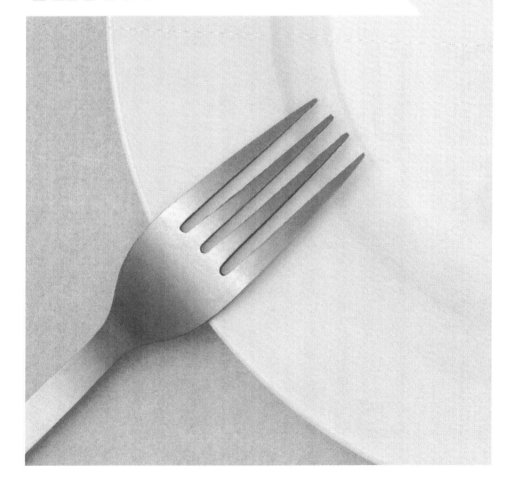

Smart Food Choices

Don't let living with diabetes overwhelm you, because it doesn't have to. If you just follow a few basic rules about daily eating, you should have no problem managing your blood sugar. Some of this information may not be new to you. But read through this section anyway: it may contain the crucial bit of information you need to make cooking and planning your meals a little easier.

- Keep your blood sugar steady by eating smaller portions spread throughout the day.

- Eat less at meals and have a snack between each meal.

- Limit high-sugar foods and limit alcohol intake.

Carbohydrates

- Pay attention to your food choices. Keep track of your carbohydrate intake and the types of carbohydrates you eat. Know what you can eat. The book *Type 2 Diabetes Basics* (International Diabetes Center, 2004) presents the following guidelines for people who want to maintain weight but do little physical activity: women can eat 45 to 60 grams of carbohydrates per meal (three to four carb choices), and men can eat 60 to 75 grams of carbohydrates per meal (five to six carb choices). If you are looking to gain or lose weight or you are physically active, check with your health care provider before changing your diet.

- Substitute all or half of the white flour in recipes with whole-wheat flour. Whole-wheat flour is often the easiest choice, but almond, oat, and soy flours are also good choices. (See the desserts section for examples.)

- Choose whole-wheat or high-fiber pastas. Some brands are blends or are higher in fiber and taste just like the traditional pastas you love to eat. Low-carb or whole-grain pastas are digested more slowly and won't cause a spike in blood sugar. They also leave you feeling full longer.

- Substitute any starchy vegetable for pasta. Spaghetti squash and zucchini are tasty options.

Sugar Substitutions and Equivalents

- Replace real sugar in recipes with low-calorie or no-calorie, natural or artificial sugar substitutes. Packages often state conversion amounts, and granular sweeteners, such as Splenda or other sucralose brands, measure cup for cup like real sugar. In the case of stevia, far less is needed to substitute for sugar, so check the package and use sparingly. Conversions, including natural sweetener options, are listed on the sweetener chart on page 246.

- Note that using fruit juice, fruit purées, honey, or molasses in place of sugar is the same as using real sugar. In some recipes these sweeteners are used in conjunction with no-calorie sweeteners to help food to brown or cakes to rise. So the blends sometimes are especially preferable in baking to achieve a browning effect.

- Natural sweeteners for diabetes include stevia, xylitol, and chicory root. Other popular no-calorie sweeteners include sucralose (Splenda), aspartame (Equal), and saccharin (Sweet'N Low).

- Don't be afraid to experiment with other sugar-free options. Today's sugar-free or low-sugar pancake syrup and imitation honey taste great. If you cannot find them in your local grocery store, you can often find them online.

- Use spices and flavorings, such as cinnamon or vanilla, to impart a sweeter flavor to foods and decrease the amount of sweetener needed.

Fat and Protein

Because diabetes increases the risk of heart disease, it is important to lower your intake of fat. Start by using the following tips to eliminate unnecessary fat from recipes:

- Sauté with a nonstick vegetable spray, or make your own spray with olive or canola oil. Spraying makes it easier to use less oil.

- Use nonfat mayonnaise, nonfat sour cream, and nonfat cream cheese. Nonfat Greek yogurt is great for adding creaminess to a recipe.

- Use reduced-fat or skim cheeses. Decrease amounts of certain cheeses. Fresh cheese usually has less fat, such as part-skim mozzarella or low-fat cottage cheese.

- Decrease fats and increase flavor in recipes by using stock or broth instead of water when cooking rice and pastas. Homemade stock is the best for flavor and to avoid the high sodium in packaged broth or stock. Keep it on hand by freezing it in ice cube trays. Pop some cubes into any recipe for added flavor.

- A touch of creaminess added at the end of cooking can go a long way. You can stir in a small amount of a high-fat ingredient such as mascarpone cheese, a rich creamy Italian cheese, or crème fraîche, which is a soured cream, at the very end of cooking.

- Monounsaturated fats are heart-healthful fats. Saturated fats should be limited or avoided.

- Eat vegetarian rather than meat entrées for dinner one to two (or more) nights a week. Also, switch to lean meats, such as lean turkey breakfast sausage or fish.

- Choose lean cuts of poultry and meat. Also, regularly include fish in your diet.

- Legumes such as beans and lentils provide protein and fiber, without the fat that accompanies meat.

Salt and Sodium

- Throw away the salt shaker, or at least try to decrease the amount of salt used. Fine-grained kosher salt (not the coarse-grained variety) is great because it dissolves easily and less can be used. But regular kosher or table salt works well for all of these recipes, as does a salt substitute such as Nu-Salt. Salt is an important ingredient in cooking and baking because it enhances flavor. If you have been guilty of oversalting your food, start cutting back now for the sake of your health. And remember, foods that are cooked from scratch have far less sodium than most prepackaged or restaurant food. The latter requires high sodium as a preservative, while the former uses sodium simply for flavor.

- According to the *Dietary Guidelines for Americans*, those with diabetes should consume no more than 1,500 mg of salt per day (between 200 and 400 mg for a full meal). Consider that there are 2,000 mg of sodium in 1 teaspoon of salt, so if a recipe calls for ¾ teaspoon of salt (1,460 mg) and serves six, then each serving is approximately 243 mg. Check with your health care professional to make sure whether this range is good for you.

- Remember that some food is naturally salty, like many cheeses and canned beans. When using these ingredients, simply cut back on added salt or omit it entirely.

- Add citrus zest for flavor, especially to low-sodium foods. Use a vegetable peeler to cut wide strips that can be added for flavor to any dish. Just remember to remove the strips before serving. For other dishes, such as desserts or pastry, use a fine microplane or cheese grater.

Healthful Seasonings

- Fresh or dry herbs—it's your choice. But remember these guidelines: fresh herbs can be added during cooking or at the end, while dried herbs are more concentrated and are added during cooking. Three tablespoons of minced fresh herb equals one tablespoon of dried. Note this guideline can vary depending on the individual herb and its age. When in doubt, add more a little bit at a time, because you can always add an ingredient to a recipe, but you can't remove it.

- Store fresh herbs in the refrigerator. Either wrap them in paper towels or stand them in a glass of water, and they will stay fresh for a few days.

- To preserve fresh herbs, freeze them as herbal ice cubes. Just chop and place some in an ice cube tray along with water and add to any recipe as needed. You can also chop and bag fresh herbs. Freeze them flat in a sandwich or snack bag, and later break off what you need. Add frozen herbs to any recipe, or thaw them for sprinkling.

- Buy spices in small amounts, and buy them whole when you can. Store them in airtight containers in a cool, dark place to preserve flavor. Whole spices can be ground in a coffee or spice grinder or with a mortar and pestle right before using. Some whole spices such as cumin, fennel, and coriander seeds benefit from being toasted first and then ground. Place spices in a sauté pan over medium heat until they become fragrant, and brown them slightly to release the natural oils and bring out the flavor. Keep pushing them around the pan so they don't burn.

A Rainbow of Whole Fruits and Vegetables

Fresh, whole, nonprocessed ingredients for cooking and eating are beneficial to a diabetic diet because of their high fiber and vitamins. Even watermelon, which is considered a high-glycemic food, is good in small amounts.

- If you prefer canned vegetables, be sure to choose low- or no-salt varieties. In the case of beans, be sure to rinse them thoroughly before using them; this lowers the sodium content. In the case of fruit, fresh always is the best choice, although using unsweetened applesauce in baking recipes helps cut the fat and sugar.

- Leafy, green vegetables such as spinach, kale, and collard greens are high in fiber, iron, and calcium.

- Cruciferous vegetables such as broccoli are high in vitamin C and omega-3s.

- Purple, red, and blue grapes; cherries; and berries offer healthful, colorful options, and supply an array of vitamins and antioxidants.

- Orange vegetables such as carrots and sweet potatoes are full of nutrients, including vitamin A, magnesium, and potassium.

Less-Refined Ingredients

In addition to eating whole foods and complex carbohydrates consisting of a variety of fruits, vegetables, whole-grain breads, and whole-grain pastas, experiment with other grains, either by adding them to other dishes or serving them by themselves. For example:

- **Amaranth.** This high-protein grain can be used for breakfast.

- **Brown rice.** Compared to white rice, this rice with the bran is much healthier. It takes longer to cook but is well worth it. Also check out brown rice blends.

- **Buckwheat or kasha.** This is used in the Kasha and Cranberry–Stuffed Acorn Squash recipe.

- **Couscous.** The Vegetable Stir-Fry pairs well with couscous.

- **Quinoa.** As a whole protein, quinoa makes a wonderful side dish or is a healthful addition to a whole-grain salad.

- **Steel-cut oats.** This is even healthier than regular oatmeal, which is quite a feat. The whole grain keeps the blood sugar from spiking and takes longer to digest. Try it by making the Extra-Creamy Apple Cinnamon Steel-Cut Oatmeal recipe.

Healthful Cooking Techniques

- **Grilling.** This is a great way to cook protein without adding fat. Grilling actually draws some fat out of the meat as it drips off during cooking. Grilling meat at high temperatures increases flavor and seals in the juices, thereby removing fat without drying out the food.

- **Oven frying** (faux frying). This technique lends crispness to foods without frying them in fat. Oven frying can be done in various ways, including using egg whites to create a crispy coating for oven-baked French fries.

- **Poaching.** Eggs, salmon, chicken, pears, and other dishes can preserve their flavor and stay tender. Poaching liquid, such as water, stock, or sometimes wine or juice (for poached fruit), is heated to just under a simmer with small bubbles occasionally floating to the top of the water. Poaching is a great method to keep chicken breasts or fish from becoming dry and overcooked.

- **Roasting.** This brings out the sweetness in vegetables and flavors in meats. Roasting at high temperatures can caramelize a food, creating those tasty, deep-cooked brown bits of natural sweet flavor.

Useful Kitchen Equipment

- **Blender or food processor.** Invest in a good one for making purées, sauces, and smoothies—it is well worth the money.

- **Ginger grater.** Grate the gingerroot finely on one of these so it can be squeezed through cheesecloth for its juice. You can also use a microplane.

- **Heavy-bottomed and nonstick pans.** Good-quality sauce and sauté pans with heavy bottoms heat evenly and prevent food from sticking or getting burnt. So check that a pan is of a good weight and quality before you purchase it. Nonstick pans mean using less oil, and cleanup is always a breeze.

- **Mandoline.** This slicer is the classic tool to make perfect chips or extra-thin slices of any vegetable or fruit.

- **Microplane.** A microplane creates a fine citrus zest, softly grates cheese (grates Parmesan into full feathery tufts), grates whole nutmegs and gingerroot or garlic (à la Rachael Ray).

10 Quick and Easy Ways to Take Charge of Diabetes

It is very important for you to learn good diabetes management to drastically reduce the many potential complications that are associated with this disease, such as high blood pressure, heart disease, stroke, kidney failure, and blindness, so you can add extra healthy, active years to your life.

Living by the Numbers

It doesn't matter if you suffer from type 1 or type 2 diabetes, or if you control your diabetes with insulin, oral medication, or diet and exercise. Since there is no cure for diabetes, the way to lead a healthy life is to make a few easy adjustments in your lifestyle:

1. **Keep your blood sugar level as close to a normal (nondiabetic) level as you safely can.** As a general guideline, this means that your blood sugar level should be between 90 mg/dL and 130 mg/dL before meals, and less than 180 mg/dL two hours after starting a meal. It is important that you set your individual goals with your health care provider, but the key to staying healthy is to make sure you do not go above these levels.

2. **Check your blood sugar level regularly.** For some people this may be up to six times a day. The new glucose monitors use tiny amounts of blood that can be taken either from the finger or forearm, making it easier and painless to perform this important task.

3. **Maintain a healthful weight.** Excess weight puts a strain on your heart, keeps cholesterol high, and increases the risk of stroke and heart attack. Losing weight is one way to bring blood sugar levels down and decrease these complications, but be sure to consult with your doctor before you start to diet.

4. **Eat well and eat regularly.** Well-balanced, low-fat meals and a regular eating schedule keep your blood sugar level (and weight) under control and help you feel your best. Save the trip to the fast-food restaurant for an occasional treat.

5. **Exercise.** Even if you're not overweight, exercise helps control your blood sugar level (making the cells take glucose out of the blood) and keeps your weight and blood pressure down. Do anything that keeps you moving: run, walk, swim, bicycle, use the stairs, and park at the far end of the lot. Find an exercise you enjoy so you will look forward to doing it every day. As the commercial says, "Just do it!"

6. **Drink moderately.** Moderation means two drinks a day for men and one a day for women. A drink is a 5-ounce glass of wine, a 12-ounce light beer, or 1.5 ounces of 80-proof distilled spirits. Make sure that your medications don't require avoiding alcohol, and get your doctor's okay.

7. **Know all you can about diabetes.** Read books and diabetes magazines, and don't be afraid to ask your doctor questions.

8. **Try new recipes that cut down on sugar and carbohydrates.** People with diabetes can eat desserts and still keep blood sugar levels in their target range by learning to eat normal-size portions and substituting artificial sweeteners for most (or all) of the sugar in a recipe.

9. **Be a smart consumer whether eating in or out.** When you shop, read package labels (low in sugar may mean high in fat). In restaurants ask for calorie and fat information on menu items and don't be afraid to ask the chef to make changes (broiled instead of fried). Know which foods affect blood sugar the most.

10. **Don't smoke.** Smoking increases your odds for many diseases, including lung cancer and stroke, and it doubles the risk of dying from cardiovascular disease (the leading cause of death among people with diabetes). If you smoke, try to quit as soon as possible and talk to your doctor if you can't quit on your own.

Breakfast

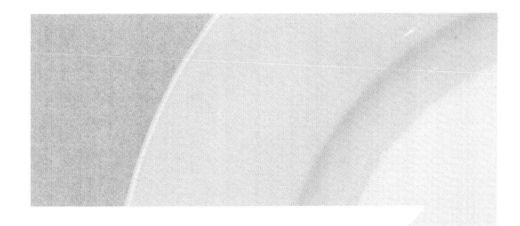

CHAPTER TWO

Breakfast

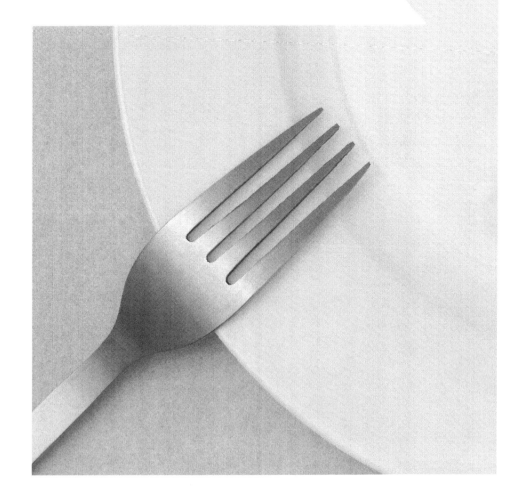

Banana Chocolate-Chip Muffins

MAKES 12 MUFFINS (1 PER SERVING)

PREPARATION TIME **10 MINUTES**
COOKING TIME **20 MINUTES**
TOTAL TIME **30 MINUTES**

Thanks to the availability of sugar substitutes, you can now enjoy these breakfast treats without worrying about your sugar levels.

This recipe works better with overripe, brown bananas. Put them in the refrigerator to brown faster.

Canola cooking spray (optional)
1½ cups sifted whole-wheat flour
2 teaspoons baking soda
½ teaspoon fine-grained kosher salt
¼ cup oat bran
Freshly grated nutmeg, to taste
¼ teaspoon ground allspice
1 cup mashed bananas
¼ cup sugarless apple butter
1 teaspoon pure vanilla extract
2 tablespoons sucralose-brown sugar blend, such as
    Splenda-brown sugar blend, or ½ teaspoon stevia powder or
    liquid concentrate, or 1 (½ teaspoon) packet stevia blends, or
    equivalent sweetener of choice
¾ cup low-fat buttermilk
2 tablespoons canola oil or olive oil (not extra-virgin)
¼ cup sugarless chocolate chips

1. Preheat the oven to 350 degrees F.

2. Line a muffin tin with papers or coat with the cooking spray.

continued ▶

3. Combine the flour, baking soda, and salt in a large bowl. Add the oat bran, nutmeg, and allspice, and stir until well combined.

4. In another bowl, add the mashed bananas, apple butter, vanilla, sweetener, buttermilk, and oil, and stir to combine.

5. Pour the wet ingredients into the flour mixture, and gently stir together to combine. Do not overmix the batter.

6. Fold in the chocolate chips;suagrs then spoon an even amount of batter into each of the muffin cups, and place the muffin tin on the middle rack of the oven.

7. Bake for about 20 minutes, or until the muffins are golden and a toothpick or paring knife inserted in the center comes out clean.

CALORIES **143**

TOTAL FAT **4 G**

CHOLESTEROL **1 MG**

SATURATED FAT **1 G**

TOTAL CARBOHYDRATES **25 G**

FIBER **2 G**

SUGAR **9 G**

SODIUM **186 MG**

PROTEIN **3 G**

Belgian Waffles with the Works

SERVES 6 (½ WAFFLE WITH ALL THE TOPPINGS PER SERVING)

PREPARATION TIME **15 MINUTES**
COOKING TIME **35 TO 45 MINUTES**
TOTAL TIME **50 MINUTES TO 1 HOUR**

This is the perfect sweet treat for that idle weekend brunch, made for someone really special. Each serving size is half a large Belgian waffle, so if you've got fewer folks, simply divide the recipe in half.

Note that the nutrition information per serving takes into account all of the toppings, some of which can be omitted.

1½ cups whole-wheat flour
2 teaspoons baking powder
½ teaspoon fine-grained kosher salt
2 tablespoons sucralose or pinch of stevia powder or drop of stevia liquid concentrate or 1 (½ teaspoon) packet stevia blends or equivalent sweetener of choice
1 egg
1¼ cups 1 percent milk, warmed
¼ cup fresh orange juice
⅓ cup unsalted butter, melted
1 sugar-free dark chocolate bar
Berry Syrup (see next page)
Whipped Cream (see next page)
Powdered Sugar (optional, see page 17)

1. Preheat your waffle iron.

2. In a bowl, whisk together the flour, baking powder, salt, and sweetener. (Note that if stevia liquid concentrate is being used, whisk with the wet ingredients in the next step, rather than here.)

3. In another bowl, whisk together the egg, milk, orange juice, and melted butter.

continued ▶

4. Mix together the wet and dry ingredients, stirring just until combined. Do not overmix the batter. It should still have some lumps.

5. Follow the manufacturer's directions for your waffle iron to prepare the waffles.

6. To make chocolate shavings, hold the bar of chocolate in one hand and use a vegetable peeler to shave the edge of the chocolate until you have ¼ cup chocolate shavings.

7. To serve, put half a waffle on a plate, top with the syrup, then whipped cream, then chocolate shavings, and finally dust with powdered sugar.

Berry Syrup

1 orange
3 cups sliced strawberries and blueberries
¼ cup stevia blends or 1 teaspoon stevia powder or stevia liquid
    concentrate or 1 cup granulated sucralose

1. Juice the orange, and remove 1- or 2-inch peels from the orange using a vegetable peeler, making sure not to leave any of the white pith on the peel, as it is bitter. (Any pith can be removed with the edge of a knife blade; a paring knife works well.)

2. In a medium saucepan with a heavy bottom, combine the orange juice and peels with the rest of the ingredients and bring to a boil. Lower the heat and simmer until the berries are soft and the syrup has thickened and reduced to half of its volume, or for about 12 to 15 minutes. The syrup is ready when it coats the back of a spoon.

Whipped Cream

1 (12-ounce) can unsweetened, nonfat evaporated milk, chilled
1 teaspoon pure vanilla extract
½ tablespoon sucralose or pinch of stevia powder (optional)

1. Pour the evaporated milk into a chilled bowl or stand-mixer bowl. Add the vanilla and the sweetener, if using.

2. Beat the chilled evaporated milk with the whisk attachment of the stand mixer or with electric beaters until stiff peaks form.

Powdered Sugar

½ cup granulated sucralose
½ teaspoon cornstarch

1. Put the sucralose and cornstarch into a blender or a food processor.

2. Mix on high speed for about 30 seconds. Scrape down the sides of the processor or blender with a rubber spatula to incorporate all of the sucralose. Blend or process on high for 30 seconds longer. Powdered sugar can be stored in a container with an airtight lid for up to 1 month.

CALORIES **323**

TOTAL FAT **12 G**

CHOLESTEROL **58 MG**

SATURATED FAT **7 G**

TOTAL CARBOHYDRATES **44 G**

FIBER **3 G**

SUGAR **16 G**

SODIUM **200 MG**

PROTEIN **11 G**

Make It a Full Meal

Because these waffles are so rich, a half waffle could be served with a simple side. Here are some options for a sumptuous brunch:

- A side salad—mixed spring greens, mesclun, or baby spinach that has been dressed with a squeeze of orange juice, a sprinkle of salt, and a drizzle of with olive oil

- A vegetable—blanched asparagus with a squeeze of lemon or orange and a sprinkle of almond slices

- Fruit—fresh berries or grapefruit slices

- Eggs—1 egg per serving, whether it's poached, fried, over easy, hard-boiled, or scrambled, with sautéed spinach

Breakfast Burrito with Spinach and Black Bean Salsa

PREPARATION TIME **15 MINUTES**
COOKING TIME **10 TO 15 MINUTES**
TOTAL TIME **25 TO 30 MINUTES**

This is a surefire favorite for a handheld breakfast on the go. Just be sure to bring the napkins, because this burrito is overstuffed with Southwestern flavor and can get a little messy.

The avocado in this recipe adds a significant amount of monounsaturated fat, a heart-healthful kind of plant fat that is easily burned as fuel by the body. If you're looking to cut down on the fat and cholesterol, try using an egg substitute or egg whites for the scramble, if desired.

1 (10-ounce) package prewashed baby spinach
1 cup low-sodium canned black beans, drained and rinsed
1 beefsteak or hothouse or 2 plum (also called Italian Roma) tomatoes, finely chopped
1 red bell pepper, cored, seeded, and finely chopped
1 tablespoon fresh lime juice
½ jalapeño, finely chopped
¼ cup chopped cilantro or parsley leaves
¼ cup chopped red onion
1 medium avocado, peeled, pitted, and chopped
6 eggs
2 tablespoons nonfat half-and-half
Olive oil or canola oil cooking spray
⅓ cup grated reduced-fat cheddar cheese
6 (10-inch) whole-wheat tortillas (burrito-size)
¼ cup nonfat sour cream
Fine-grained kosher salt, to taste

1. Wilt the spinach by adding the entire bag and ¼ cup of water to a sauté pan. Cook over medium-low heat, covered, to steam for about 5 minutes.

Press with the back of a spoon through a strainer to remove any excess water, and put the spinach on a covered plate.

2. In a medium bowl, combine the beans, tomato, bell pepper, lime juice, jalapeño, cilantro or parsley, onion, and avocado to make a bean salsa. Set aside.

3. Whisk the eggs with the nonfat half-and-half until well combined.

4. Coat a sauté pan with an even layer of oil or cooking spray, and place over medium heat. Add the eggs and stir constantly for about 3 to 5 minutes for a soft scramble.

5. Remove from the heat, top with grated cheddar, cover, and let stand for 1 minute.

6. Add a thin layer of an even amount of eggs to 6 wraps. Top with the bean salsa and sour cream, and season with salt. Roll to wrap, tucking in the ends, before serving.

CALORIES **357**

FIBER **8 G**

TOTAL FAT **15 G**

SUGAR **2 G**

CHOLESTEROL **170 MG**

SODIUM **250 MG**

SATURATED FAT **4 G**

PROTEIN **15 G**

TOTAL CARBOHYDRATES **40 G**

Buckwheat Buttermilk Pancakes with Homemade Applesauce

SERVES 6

PREPARATION TIME **10 MINUTES**
COOKING TIME **30 TO 40 MINUTES**
TOTAL TIME **40 TO 50 MINUTES**

These pancakes are hearty and filling, and they will really hit the spot on a chilly winter morning. Be sure to use high-quality butter; it'll really make a big difference.

Homemade applesauce is easy to make. Note that the sweetener is optional on the applesauce, and it is not recommended if cooking the apples in cider or juice, as that will already make your sauce sweeter. If using water, taste for sweetness. If it's needed, stir in a little sweetener toward the end of the cooking time.

1½ cups buckwheat flour
3 tablespoons sucralose, or ⅛ teaspoon stevia powder or stevia liquid concentrate, or ½ packet (¼ teaspoon) stevia blends
½ teaspoon fine-grained kosher salt
1 teaspoon baking soda
3 tablespoons unsalted butter, melted
2 cups buttermilk, divided
1 egg
Canola oil cooking spray
Applesauce (see next page)

1. In a large bowl, mix together the flour, sweetener, salt, and baking soda until well combined. Gradually pour in the melted butter, whisking constantly as you add it.

2. In a separate bowl, whisk together half of the buttermilk and the egg until combined. Whisk the mixture into the dry ingredients. Add the remaining buttermilk slowly, pouring and whisking until you achieve the desired consistency. Only whisk lightly to combine, and do not overmix. Some lumps are fine.

3. Heat a griddle, cast-iron skillet, or nonstick pan on medium heat, and coat with the cooking spray.

4. Use a small ladle to pour a small amount of batter into the pan; then gently swirl the batter with the bottom of the ladle to make a more perfect circle on the hot griddle.

5. Turn down the heat to medium-low. Cook for 2 to 3 minutes on one side, until bubbles form on the surface of the pancake.

6. Using a heatproof rubber spatula, gently loosen the edges and flip the pancake.

7. Cook for another 1 to 2 minutes, or until nicely browned.

8. Keep the pancakes warm as you make more batches by putting them on a covered plate in the oven on the lowest setting. Spray more oil on the pan between each batch of pancakes.

9. To serve, stack 3 layers of pancakes, with a layer of applesauce between each layer and over the stack.

Applesauce

3 McIntosh, Golden Delicious, or Granny Smith apples, peeled, cored, and chopped into bite-size pieces
1 cinnamon stick or 1 teaspoon ground cinnamon
¼ cup water or apple cider or apple juice
½ tablespoon sucralose or 1 drop of liquid stevia or ¼ packet (⅛ teaspoon) stevia blends (optional)

1. Bring the apples, cinnamon, and cider just to a boil in a heavy-bottomed medium saucepan. When they reach a boil, stir, reduce heat to low, and cover.

2. Cook for 10 minutes and taste. Add a sweetener, if desired, and additional cider, if necessary. Continue to cook for 10 minutes. Remove the cinnamon stick, if using, before serving.

CALORIES **263**	FIBER **5 G**
TOTAL FAT **12 G**	SUGAR **13 G**
CHOLESTEROL **46 MG**	SODIUM **250 MG**
SATURATED FAT **5 G**	PROTEIN **7 G**
TOTAL CARBOHYDRATES **36 G**	

Eggs Florentine with Yogurt Hollandaise Sauce

SERVES 4 (1 EGG AND ½ MUFFIN PER SERVING)

PREPARATION TIME **10 MINUTES**
COOKING TIME **10 MINUTES**
TOTAL TIME **20 MINUTES**

Perfectly poached eggs with runny centers, wilted baby spinach, and a yogurt hollandaise sauce come together to make a great eggs Florentine.

For a traditional eggs Benedict dish, just replace the spinach with bacon or smoked salmon. (But be sure to take into account the change to the nutritional value of the dish.)

1 (10-ounce) package prewashed baby spinach
1 cup low-fat Greek yogurt
Pinch of ground turmeric
Juice of ½ lemon
Pinch of cayenne pepper (optional)
Fine-grained kosher salt, to taste
2 teaspoons white vinegar
4 eggs
2 whole-wheat English muffins, split in half
1 tablespoon unsalted butter

1. Wilt the spinach by adding the entire bag and ¼ cup of water to a sauté pan. Cook over medium-low heat, covered, to steam for about 5 minutes. Press with the back of a spoon through a strainer to remove any excess water, and put spinach on a covered plate.

2. In a medium bowl, whisk together the yogurt and turmeric until well combined, and then add in the lemon juice and stir. Stir in cayenne pepper, if desired. Season with salt.

3. To poach the eggs, fill a medium sauté pan two-thirds full with water and add the vinegar. Over medium-high heat, bring the water to a low simmer, and then crack one egg at a time, add it to a small cup, and then slide it onto the surface of the water. (Do not drop the eggs in from above.) Nudge

the egg white with a spoon to keep it close to the yolk and prevent it from spreading out in the water.

4. When one egg begins to firm slightly, slip in the next egg, until all the eggs are in the pan. Gently remove from the heat, cover the pan, and allow the eggs to sit for 3 to 4 minutes or so, until they're done. Then remove them carefully with a slotted spoon.

5. Toast and butter the English muffin halves. Top each one with the spinach and then a poached egg, and pour some yogurt hollandaise over the top.

CALORIES **155**

TOTAL FAT **8 G**

CHOLESTEROL **175 MG**

SATURATED FAT **4 G**

TOTAL CARBOHYDRATES **10 G**

FIBER **1 G**

SUGAR **5 G**

SODIUM **639 MG**

PROTEIN **10 G**

Extra-Creamy Apple Cinnamon Steel-Cut Oatmeal

SERVES 4

PREPARATION TIME **10 MINUTES (PLUS OVERNIGHT IN REFRIGERATOR)**
COOKING TIME **15 MINUTES**
TOTAL TIME **25 MINUTES (PLUS OVERNIGHT IN REFRIGERATOR)**

Steel-cut oats are a more nutritious, less-processed version of oatmeal, and the additional time needed for cooking is well worth their nutty flavor and chewier texture.

Using the half-and-half will make for an extra-rich and creamy dish; if, however, you prefer a lower-fat version, replace the half-and-half with two more cups of milk.

1 cup steel-cut oats
2 cups 1 percent milk
2 cups nonfat half-and-half
2 cinnamon sticks or 1 teaspoon ground cinnamon
1 McIntosh, Granny Smith, or Golden Delicious apple, peeled, cored, and diced
⅛ teaspoon fine-grained kosher salt
1 teaspoon pure vanilla extract
¼ cup dried cranberries or raisins, divided
3 tablespoons sucralose-brown sugar blend or 1 packet stevia blends or ½ teaspoon stevia or equivalent sweetener of choice (optional)
½ cup chopped walnuts

1. In a medium bowl, combine the oats, milk, and half-and-half, and cover. Soak in the refrigerator overnight.

2. Remove the oats from the refrigerator, and place into a heavy-bottomed saucepan. Add the cinnamon, diced apples, and salt, and bring to a boil over high heat.

3. Stir and reduce the heat to medium-low. Simmer, stirring often, until the oatmeal is soft, for about 10 minutes.

4. Stir in the vanilla, half the cranberries or raisins, and the sweetener, if using. Simmer for 5 minutes more, stirring continuously. Remove the cinnamon sticks, if using.

5. Meanwhile, in a separate sauté pan, toast the chopped walnuts over medium heat for 6 minutes, stirring, until golden and fragrant.

6. Spoon the oatmeal into bowls. Sprinkle with the remaining cranberries or raisins and with the toasted walnuts.

CALORIES **287**

TOTAL FAT **11 G**

CHOLESTEROL **10 MG**

SATURATED FAT **2 G**

TOTAL CARBOHYDRATES **38 G**

FIBER **4 G**

SUGAR **15 G**

SODIUM **94 MG**

PROTEIN **11 G**

Parmesan and Asparagus Frittata

SERVES 6

PREPARATION TIME **10 MINUTES**
COOKING TIME **15 TO 20 MINUTES**
TOTAL TIME **25 TO 30 MINUTES**

If you aren't familiar with this dish, think of it a kind of quiche, except a little firmer and without a crust. Frittatas make for a hearty breakfast or can be served with simply dressed mixed greens for brunch.

2 lean turkey or chicken sausages
1 tablespoon extra-virgin olive oil
¼ cup chopped roasted asparagus
¼ cup chopped red bell pepper
1 chopped plum tomato
6 eggs, scrambled
2 tablespoons nonfat half-and-half
½ cup grated Parmesan, divided
⅛ teaspoon fine-grained kosher salt
⅛ teaspoon freshly ground black pepper

1. Preheat the oven to broil setting.

2. Remove the casings from the turkey or chicken sausage, and crumble the meat in a medium sauté pan. Cook thoroughly over medium-high heat. Set aside.

3. Heat a nonstick, oven-safe sauté pan, skillet, or griddle pan over medium-high heat. Add the olive oil to the pan. Add the asparagus, bell pepper, and tomato, and cook for about 3 to 5 minutes.

4. Meanwhile, whisk the eggs, half-and-half, ¼ cup of the Parmesan, salt, and pepper in a medium bowl.

5. Add the egg mixture and sausage crumbles to the pan with the vegetables. Cook for 5 minutes, or until the egg mixture has set on the bottom and begins to firm up on top.

6. Top with the remaining Parmesan. Place pan in the oven, and broil for 3 to 4 minutes, until golden and firm. Remove the frittata from the oven, cut it into 6 slices, and serve hot.

CALORIES **255**

TOTAL FAT **15 G**

CHOLESTEROL **224 MG**

SATURATED FAT **5 G**

TOTAL CARBOHYDRATES **2 G**

FIBER **0 G**

SUGAR **1 G**

SODIUM **200 MG**

PROTEIN **27 G**

"AB&J" French Toast

SERVES 6 (1 PIECE OF STUFFED FRENCH TOAST PER SERVING)

PREPARATION TIME **10 MINUTES**
COOKING TIME **25 MINUTES**
TOTAL TIME **35 MINUTES**

The A in the title is for "almond"—almond butter makes for a fresher, more adult version of the universally loved PB&J sandwich (though you can also use peanut or walnut butter). Here you take this idea a step further, and turn a plain sandwich into syrup-smothered French toast.

Roasting the almonds increases their flavor. Using the warm nuts helps them release their oils and form a paste faster. For best results, follow the recipe below to make your fresh almond butter. However, if you need to save time, almond butter can be purchased and used straight from the jar. Just choose one that is 100 percent natural and unsweetened.

1 cup almonds
1 teaspoon walnut, almond, or canola oil
Fine-grained kosher salt, to taste
2 eggs
½ cup milk
¼ teaspoon pure vanilla extract
⅛ teaspoon ground cinnamon
12 slices whole-wheat bread
1 cup sliced strawberries or sliced bananas (or a mix of both)
2 tablespoons unsalted butter, for cooking
Berry Syrup (see page 16)

1. Start by preparing the almond butter (skip this step if you're planning to use store-bought). Roast the almonds on the stove top in a heavy-bottomed sauté pan or a skillet over medium-high heat. Stir frequently for 5 to 8 minutes until golden brown and fragrant. Do not allow the nuts to burn.

2. Put the hot roasted nuts directly into the food processor, and pulse on high speed.

3. Stop periodically to scrape down the sides with a rubber spatula. Add the oil in a drizzle while the processor is running. Add a sprinkle of salt, and empty the almond butter into a small bowl.

4. Next, prepare the French toast. In a small bowl, whisk together the eggs, milk, vanilla, and cinnamon. Spread the almond butter in a thin layer on one side of all of the bread slices. Layer the slices of fruit on top of the almond butter on 6 of the slices.

5. Put the remaining bread slices on top of the slices with fruit to form sandwiches, and press the edges all around to seal in the filling.

6. Melt the butter on a griddle or in a pan over medium-low heat. Carefully dip the stuffed French toast in the egg mixture, and flip to coat both sides evenly. Let excess egg drip back into the bowl.

7. Cook for 2 to 3 minutes on one side; then flip and repeat on the other side until the French toast has firmed and is golden brown in color. Serve with Berry Syrup.

CALORIES **401**

TOTAL FAT **18 G**

CHOLESTEROL **58 MG**

SATURATED FAT **3 G**

TOTAL CARBOHYDRATES **46 G**

FIBER **10 G**

SUGAR **13 G**

SODIUM **693 MG**

PROTEIN **18 G**

Breakfast Turkey Sausage Patties

MAKES 8 PATTIES (1 PER SERVING)

PREPARATION TIME **5 MINUTES**
COOKING TIME **10 MINUTES**
TOTAL TIME **15 MINUTES**

This turkey breakfast sausage is much better than what can be purchased in the store. The fennel seed is the key ingredient that gives this sausage a distinct flavor. If you like your sausage extra spicy, just add extra chili flakes.

You can serve turkey sausage as a side or in a breakfast sandwich. To use it as an entrée, increase the serving size to two patties per person. Note that this is a no-carbohydrate, high-protein food.

1 pound lean ground turkey
½ teaspoon dried sage
¼ teaspoon ground ginger
1 teaspoon fennel seeds
¼ teaspoon red chili flakes (optional)
1 teaspoon fine-grained kosher salt
½ teaspoon freshly ground black pepper
Canola oil cooking spray

1. Crumble the turkey into a large bowl. Add the rest of the ingredients, except for the cooking spray, and mix well with your hands, dispersing the spices evenly. Shape into 8 patties.

2. In a nonstick skillet coated with the cooking spray, cook the sausage patties over medium heat for about 5 minutes on each side until they are firm.

CALORIES **82**
TOTAL FAT **5 G**
CHOLESTEROL **49 MG**
SATURATED FAT **1 G**
TOTAL CARBOHYDRATES **0 G**

FIBER **0 G**
SUGAR **0 G**
SODIUM **200 MG**
PROTEIN **10 G**

Velvety Cheese Grits

SERVES 4

PREPARATION TIME **5 MINUTES**
COOKING TIME **5 MINUTES**
TOTAL TIME **10 MINUTES**

This quick version of the Southern favorite is so tasty and smooth that it can be summed up as a warm bowl of comfort. You can eat a bowl of grits for breakfast, but it works just as well as a side during dinnertime.

1 cup nonfat half-and-half
2 cups low-sodium chicken stock or water
½ cup quick-cooking grits
8 tablespoons grated reduced-fat extra-sharp cheddar cheese,
    2 tablespoons reserved
1 tablespoon unsalted butter
Fine-grained kosher salt and freshly ground black pepper, to taste
2 tablespoons nonfat sour cream or yogurt
1 teaspoon hot sauce of choice (optional)

1. In a medium saucepan over high heat, combine the half-and-half and stock. Bring the mixture to a rapid simmer (almost until boiling). Reduce the heat to low, and gradually add in the grits a little at a time, whisking constantly until they start to thicken, or for about 5 to 6 minutes.

2. Remove the pan from the heat, and whisk in the cheese and butter. Cover and let stand until most of the liquid has been absorbed and the grits are creamy, for about 3 minutes.

3. Stir in the sour cream or yogurt, and the hot sauce, if using. Serve sprinkled with the reserved 2 tablespoons of cheese.

CALORIES **208**	FIBER **1 G**
TOTAL FAT **3 G**	SUGAR **3 G**
CHOLESTEROL **24 MG**	SODIUM **229 MG**
SATURATED FAT **1 G**	PROTEIN **9 G**
TOTAL CARBOHYDRATES **24 G**	

Small Bites

Classic Deviled Eggs

Arancini: Cheesy Risotto Balls
with a Crisp Crust

Baked Mozzarella Sticks with
Fresh Marinara Sauce

Crisp Parmesan Tuiles with a
Tapenade Dollop

Miniature Lobster Rolls

Grilled Cheeseburger Sliders

Oven-Fried Buffalo Wings with
Blue Cheese Dip

Pigs in a Blanket with Cheddar
Cheese Sauce

Sweet and Savory
Swedish Meatballs

Smoked Salmon on Crostini

Small Bites

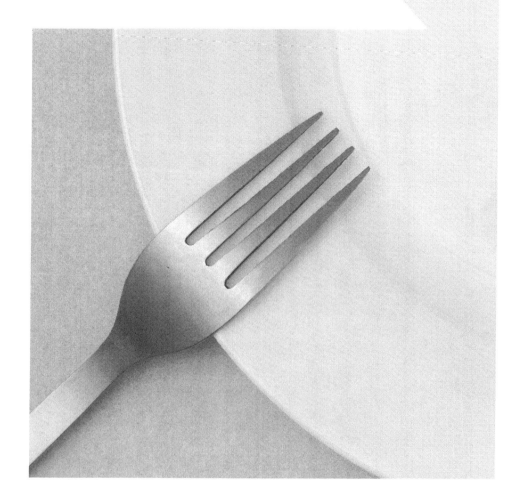

Classic Deviled Eggs

SERVES 6

PREPARATION TIME **5 MINUTES**
COOKING TIME **15 MINUTES**
TOTAL TIME **20 MINUTES**

Deviled eggs is a classic party dish, particularly popular in the South. Note that two deviled egg halves make a serving, so this recipe serves six. For larger get-togethers, use at least a dozen eggs to serve twelve people.

6 eggs
1 teaspoon fine-grained kosher salt, plus more, to taste
1 tablespoon plus 1 teaspoon white vinegar, divided
¼ cup low-fat or nonfat mayonnaise
1 teaspoon yellow mustard
Freshly ground black pepper, to taste
½ teaspoon ground paprika for garnish
¼ cup minced chives for garnish (optional)

1. Put the eggs in an even layer in a pot, covered by 2 inches of cold water, 1 teaspoon of the salt, and 1 tablespoon of the white vinegar. Cook on high heat until the water is just about to boil; then remove them from the heat, cover, and let sit for 12 minutes in the hot water.

2. Remove the eggs with a slotted spoon, and place them in a bowl of ice water.

3. Carefully crack the eggs to remove the shells and peels.

4. Halve the eggs lengthwise, spooning out the yolks and placing them in a bowl. Place the whites on a plate or your serving tray. Mash the yolks with a potato masher or a fork. Add the remaining vinegar, the mayonnaise, and the mustard, and stir to combine. Season with salt and pepper.

5. Fill the egg whites with 1 tablespoon of the deviled yolks. Garnish with a sprinkle of paprika and with chives, if desired.

CALORIES **148**
TOTAL FAT **14 G**
CHOLESTEROL **164 MG**
SATURATED FAT **3 G**
TOTAL CARBOHYDRATES **1 G**

FIBER **0 G**
SUGAR **0 G**
SODIUM **131 MG**
PROTEIN **6 G**

Arancini: Cheesy Risotto Balls with a Crisp Crust

SERVES 10

PREPARATION TIME **10 MINUTES**
COOKING TIME **25 TO 30 MINUTES**
TOTAL TIME **35 TO 40 MINUTES**

Risotto, or creamy short-grained rice, is delicious, and this snack was originally a way to turn leftovers into hearty Italian hors d'oeuvres. Chances are, you don't have any cooked risotto around, but not to worry—you can use short-grained brown rice and save yourself the trouble. When rolled into balls and made crisp on the outside, each bite-size morsel tastes like a decadent treat.

To serve, insert a toothpick in each arancini and include a marinara sauce dip on the side. (See Baked Mozzarella Sticks with Fresh Marinara Sauce, page 38, to make this sauce.)

1 tablespoon olive oil
¼ white onion or 2 shallots, finely chopped
1 (10-ounce) package prewashed baby spinach
2 garlic cloves, minced
1 cup short-grain instant or fast-cooking brown rice
1 cup dry white wine
1 cup mushroom, chicken, or vegetable stock
¼ cup grated Parmesan cheese
Olive oil cooking spray
All-purpose flour, for dredging
½ cup seasoned bread crumbs
⅛ cup grated Romano cheese
1 tablespoon crushed red pepper flakes
2 eggs

1. Preheat the oven to 375 degrees F.

2. Put olive oil in sauté pan over medium-high heat.

3. Add the onion and cook until softened and translucent. Add 1 tablespoon of water and the baby spinach, stir, and cover until spinach is wilted and

cooked through. Add the garlic and cook for an additional 30 seconds, until golden and fragrant. Remove from the heat.

4. Squeeze any excess liquid from the spinach; chop it on a cutting board.

5. Meanwhile, in a separate large pot, combine the uncooked brown rice, wine, and stock, and stir constantly over high heat; bring the mixture to a boil. Once boiling, stir again, reduce heat to low, cover, and let simmer for 10 to 12 minutes, until the rice is cooked. Remove from the heat, and stir in the spinach mixture until well combined.

6. Cool to room temperature. Add in the freshly grated Parmesan cheese.

7. Spray a baking sheet with olive oil cooking spray.

8. Sprinkle an even layer of flour onto a large, flat plate.

9. Combine the bread crumbs with the grated Romano cheese and red pepper flakes, and spread an even layer onto a second plate.

10. Beat the eggs together in a shallow bowl.

11. Roll the rice mixture into 1-inch balls. Dredge each ball first in the flour. Next coat with the beaten egg, then roll in the bread crumbs to coat. Place on the baking sheet. Repeat with the remaining balls.

12. Spray the arancini with a light layer of olive oil cooking spray.

13. Bake for 12 to 15 minutes, or until the arancini turn golden-brown. Serve hot.

Small Bites

CALORIES **165**

TOTAL FAT **5 G**

CHOLESTEROL **36 MG**

SATURATED FAT **1 G**

TOTAL CARBOHYDRATES **21 G**

FIBER **2 G**

SUGAR **1 G**

SODIUM **191 MG**

PROTEIN **6 G**

Baked Mozzarella Sticks with Fresh Marinara Sauce

SERVES 4

PREPARATION TIME **15 MINUTES**
COOKING TIME **5 TO 10 MINUTES**
TOTAL TIME **20 TO 25 MINUTES**

You don't need a deep fryer to make these addictive mozzarella sticks; bread-ing and baking melts them on the inside and forms a deliciously crisp crust on the outside. The marinara sauce has been factored into the nutrition informa-tion. It makes the perfect dip. (Use it with Arancini on page 36, too.)

Olive oil cooking spray
1 (8-ounce) package reduced-fat or part-skim mozzarella cheese
2 tablespoons all-purpose flour
2 egg whites
½ cup plain or whole-wheat panko bread crumbs
1 tablespoon extra-virgin olive oil
1 (15-ounce) can crushed tomatoes (fire-roasted preferred), strained
½ teaspoon fresh thyme
½ teaspoon dried oregano
1 tablespoon balsamic vinegar (optional)
3 garlic cloves, minced
Fine-grained kosher salt and freshly ground black pepper, to taste
2 tablespoons chopped fresh parsley for garnish (optional)

1. Preheat the oven to 400 degrees F. Coat a baking sheet evenly with the cooking spray.

2. Cut the mozzarella block in half, and then cut each half into four sticks.

3. Place the flour in a thin layer on a plate. Place the egg whites in a small bowl. Cover a second plate with an even layer of bread crumbs. Dip the moz-zarella sticks first in the flour to coat, then into the egg whites, and then into the bread crumbs, turning and pressing the cheese down to coat completely.

4. After each piece of cheese is coated, carefully place it on the baking sheet. Spray the tops with a light, even layer of the cooking spray. Bake for 5 min-utes, until golden brown.

5. Meanwhile, prepare the marinara sauce. In a sauté pan over medium-high heat, heat the olive oil until shimmering; add the crushed tomatoes, thyme, oregano, and balsamic vinegar, if using, and cook until hot. Add the minced garlic, and cook for an additional 30 seconds, or until the garlic is golden and fragrant but not burnt.

6. Remove mozzarella sticks from the heat, and season with salt and pepper. Spoon the marinara over the mozzarella sticks and serve. Sprinkle with parsley as garnish, if desired.

CALORIES **141**

TOTAL FAT **6 G**

CHOLESTEROL **10 MG**

SATURATED FAT **2 G**

TOTAL CARBOHYDRATES **13 G**

FIBER **4 G**

SUGAR **6 G**

SODIUM **240 MG**

PROTEIN **9 G**

Small Bites

Crisp Parmesan Tuiles with a Tapenade Dollop

SERVES 8

PREPARATION TIME **10 MINUTES**
COOKING TIME **10 TO 12 MINUTES**
TOTAL TIME **20 TO 22 MINUTES**

These tuiles, or delicate thin crisps, are made with one ingredient—Parmesan—and topped with an easy-to-make light tapenade. Make sure you use fresh basil in this recipe; it gives the tapenade a really fresh taste.

2 cups freshly grated Parmesan cheese
1 cup jarred roasted red peppers, drained and sliced
1 plum (or Italian Roma) tomato, finely chopped
5 kalamata olives, chopped
5 fresh basil leaves, finely chopped
Fine-grained kosher salt and freshly ground black pepper, to taste

1. Preheat the oven to 350 degrees F.

2. Line a baking sheet with parchment or waxed paper. Use about 3 tablespoons of the grated cheese to make 3-inch circles; continue until all the cheese is used up and the tuiles are evenly spread out. Bake for about 10 to 12 minutes, until golden brown.

3. The warm tuiles can be left flat or be shaped into taco-like shapes by placing and pressing them gently over a rolling pin. Allow the crisps to cool on the rolling pin, and then slide off to remove.

4. Just prior to serving the tuiles, assemble the topping by combining the rest of the ingredients in a small bowl.

5. Press the mixture with a small spoon to extract any juice. Add a small teaspoon of the topping (no juice or sauce) to the top of each tuile, and serve immediately.

CALORIES **143**
TOTAL FAT **9 G**
CHOLESTEROL **22 MG**
SATURATED FAT **5 G**
TOTAL CARBOHYDRATES **3 G**

FIBER **1 G**
SUGAR **2 G**
SODIUM **220 MG**
PROTEIN **12 G**

Miniature Lobster Rolls

SERVES 12 (2 MINIATURE LOBSTER ROLLS PER SERVING)

PREPARATION TIME **10 MINUTES**
COOKING TIME **2 TO 3 MINUTES**
TOTAL TIME **12 TO 13 MINUTES**

Whip up these lobster rolls at the next festive occasion. Toasting the rolls with butter is the traditional way to serve them. If top-split hot dog rolls cannot be found, it's okay to use the traditional ones that are side cut.

3½ cups cooked lobster meat, finely chopped
½ cup nonfat mayonnaise
Juice of ½ lemon
3 tablespoons finely chopped fresh chives, divided
½ teaspoon Old Bay 30 percent less sodium seasoning
2 tablespoons unsalted butter, chopped into small pieces
8 whole-wheat top-split hot dog buns or regular whole-wheat
    hot dog buns, each cut in 3 even-size pieces

1. In a medium or large bowl, combine the lobster meat, mayonnaise, lemon juice, 2 tablespoons of the chives, and seasoning.

2. In a sauté pan over medium heat, melt the butter pieces. Add the hot dog buns facedown to toast until golden, for about 2 to 3 minutes each.

3. Place the hot dog buns on a platter, spoon in the lobster mixture, and sprinkle with the remaining 1 tablespoon of chives to garnish.

CALORIES **153**
TOTAL FAT **11 G**
CHOLESTEROL **53 MG**
SATURATED FAT **3 G**
TOTAL CARBOHYDRATES **7 G**

FIBER **0 G**
SUGAR **1 G**
SODIUM **271 MG**
PROTEIN **8 G**

Small Bites

Grilled Cheeseburger Sliders

SERVES 12 (1 SLIDER PER SERVING)

PREPARATION TIME **10 MINUTES**
COOKING TIME **15 MINUTES**
TOTAL TIME **25 MINUTES**

Miniature burgers are delicious as a snack or hors d'oeuvres. The recipe that follows makes enough for twelve, but you can divide it to make less for fewer folks. Don't forget, if you use condiments, they may affect the nutritional content of the overall dish.

When cooking burgers, it's important not to press or poke them, to keep the meat juices in. When the burgers are done, they need to sit and "rest," which allows the juices to settle and the meat to actually continue cooking a little bit more. That makes for a better-tasting burger, so be patient.

1 pound lean ground turkey or lean ground sirloin
1½ tablespoons Worcestershire sauce
¼ teaspoon finely grained kosher salt
½ teaspoon freshly ground black pepper
Canola oil cooking spray
½ cup reduced-fat shredded sharp or extra-sharp cheddar cheese
12 miniature whole-wheat buns or whole-wheat dinner rolls
2 dill pickles, cut into thin slices

1. In a bowl, combine the ground meat, Worcestershire sauce, salt, and pepper, using your hands to massage the ingredients into the meat evenly. Form 12 even-size balls and then flatten them into patties, smoothing edges if necessary.

2. Oil the grates of a grill, grill pan, or cast-iron skillet with the cooking spray. (If the grill or stove top is on, do not spray directly onto grates or pan; spray onto a paper towel. Holding the towel with kitchen tongs, apply the spray to the cooking surface until well coated.)

3. Spray each meat patty with oil on both sides. Cook the burgers over medium heat, for 2 minutes per side, using tongs or a spatula to flip, and top with shredded cheese after 1 minute on the second side. When the burgers reach 160 degrees F, let them sit on a covered plate.

4. Meanwhile, spray buns with cooking spray and place facedown on the grill, cooking for 30 seconds to 1 minute, just until golden and crisp on the inside.

5. Place the burgers on grilled buns with pickle slices.

CALORIES **147**

TOTAL FAT **8 G**

CHOLESTEROL **38 MG**

SATURATED FAT **2 G**

TOTAL CARBOHYDRATES **11 G**

FIBER **2 G**

SUGAR **2 G**

SODIUM **307 MG**

PROTEIN **10 G**

Oven-Fried Buffalo Wings with Blue Cheese Dip

SERVES 6

PREPARATION TIME **35 MINUTES (INCLUDING 30 MINUTES MARINATING TIME)**
COOKING TIME **55 MINUTES TO 1 HOUR**
TOTAL TIME **2 HOURS 5 MINUTES (INCLUDING 30 MINUTES MARINATING TIME)**

This recipe calls for whole chicken wings, which you can cleave at the bone and then slice off the pointy tips of the wings. This method can save money, since it's often cheaper to buy a pound of whole wings than already-cut buffalo wings. However, to save time, you can just purchase split chicken wings, or drumettes.

1 pound chicken wings
Fine-grained kosher salt and freshly ground black pepper, to taste
1 tablespoon unsalted butter
5 garlic cloves, minced
⅓ cup hot sauce
½ cup reduced-fat blue cheese crumbles
1 cup nonfat Greek yogurt
Canola oil cooking spray

1. Split the wings at the joint to separate them into drumettes and wing tips, and place them into a bowl. Sprinkle with salt and pepper.

2. In a sauté pan over low heat, melt the butter. Add the garlic and cook for 30 seconds until it is golden and fragrant but not burnt. Stir in the hot sauce immediately until well combined.

3. Pour the hot sauce mixture over the wings, and coat thoroughly. Cover the bowl, and put in the refrigerator for at least 30 minutes to marinate.

4. Meanwhile, make the dip by mixing together the blue cheese and Greek yogurt in a small bowl until well combined. Cover and refrigerate.

5. Preheat the oven to 375 degrees F, and spray a baking dish with cooking spray.

6. Put the chicken wings in the baking dish and bake for 30 minutes. After 30 minutes, flip the wings, and baste the other side with the hot sauce marinade.

7. Bake for 25 to 30 minutes more. Check the wings periodically, and add more sauce now and then with the basting brush.

8. Remove the wings from the oven, and allow them to cool on the stove top. Baste with the marinade and juices.

9. Serve with the blue cheese dip.

CALORIES **255**

TOTAL FAT **18 G**

CHOLESTEROL **74 MG**

SATURATED FAT **7 G**

TOTAL CARBOHYDRATES **5 G**

FIBER **0 G**

SUGAR **3 G**

SODIUM **580 MG**

PROTEIN **19 G**

Pigs in a Blanket with Cheddar Cheese Sauce

SERVES 10

PREPARATION TIME **15 MINUTES**
COOKING TIME **15 MINUTES**
TOTAL TIME **30 MINUTES**

Kids love these and so do their parents, aunts, and uncles. If you want to lighten up the sauce, serve the pigs in a blanket with a simple mustard dip instead. Dijon, yellow, or brown spicy mustard would all be good. Some people like to mix the mustard with nonfat mayonnaise for a creamier-style dip.

8 reduced-fat hot dogs of choice
2 tablespoons all-purpose flour, divided
2 tubes reduced-fat crescent roll dough
1 tablespoon olive oil
1 cup 1 percent milk
Pinch of freshly grated nutmeg
½ cup reduced-fat sharp cheddar cheese
1 tablespoon yellow or Dijon mustard (optional)
Fine-grained kosher salt and freshly ground white pepper
    (optional), to taste

1. Preheat the oven to 375 degrees F.

2. Cut each hot dog into quarters to make 4 even pieces. Set aside.

3. Sprinkle 1 tablespoon of the flour on a cutting board. Open the crescent tubes and separate the dough triangles, stretching each triangle a little to make it a little larger. Then place them on the floured cutting board.

4. Cut each triangle in half. Placing a hot dog piece at the base of each triangle, roll it up until the point of the triangle wraps around the center.

5. On an ungreased baking sheet, line up the pigs in a blanket in an even layer so that they are not touching and have some space in between.

6. Cook for about 10 to 15 minutes, or until the dough is golden brown on the outside and cooked through.

7. Meanwhile, make the cheese sauce. In the bottom of a saucepan, over medium-high heat, whisk the olive oil and the remaining flour constantly until it reaches a golden hue and has a nutty fragrance, for about 3 to 5 minutes. Do not stop whisking, or this olive oil roux will burn.

8. With the heat on medium, slowly drizzle in the milk, whisking constantly and briskly the whole time. The sauce should become the consistency of a very thick cream. This is the béchamel sauce. The nutmeg can be grated directly into the sauce or measured out. Use the side of a box grater, a nutmeg or spice grater, or a microplane. If grating the nutmeg directly into the sauce, 1 or 2 scrapes equal a pinch.

9. Remove from the heat, and then whisk in the grated cheddar. Stir in the mustard, if using, and combine well. Season with salt and pepper.

10. Serve the cheddar cheese sauce in a small bowl alongside the pigs in a blanket.

CALORIES **138**

TOTAL FAT **9 G**

CHOLESTEROL **28 MG**

SATURATED FAT **4 G**

TOTAL CARBOHYDRATES **7 G**

FIBER **0 G**

SUGAR **0 G**

SODIUM **278 MG**

PROTEIN **8 G**

Sweet and Savory Swedish Meatballs

SERVES 6

PREPARATION TIME **20 MINUTES**
COOKING TIME **15 TO 20 MINUTES**
TOTAL TIME **35 TO 40 MINUTES**

Swedish meatballs are a great appetizer, and this recipe makes enough for six, but you can also turn them into a meal for fewer people. Try serving them over mashed parsnips and celery root, over mashed cauliflower, or even with brown rice or egg noodles.

1 large white onion, grated finely with a cheese grater
⅓ cup whole-wheat bread crumbs
¾ teaspoon fine-grained kosher salt, divided
2 tablespoons olive oil, divided
½ teaspoon freshly ground black pepper
¼ teaspoon freshly grated nutmeg
⅛ teaspoon ground allspice
¼ teaspoon ground cardamom
½ pound ground pork
½ pound lean ground turkey
½ pound button mushrooms, sliced
½ lemon
¼ cup all-purpose flour
1 (14-ounce) can reduced-sodium chicken stock
½ cup nonfat sour cream
1 tablespoon lingonberry, red currant, blackberry, or
    black currant jam
¼ cup finely chopped fresh parsley

1. Combine the onion, bread crumbs, ¼ teaspoon of the salt, 1 tablespoon of the olive oil, black pepper, nutmeg, allspice, and cardamom in a large bowl. Add the ground pork and turkey, and combine thoroughly. Use the ground meat to form about 20 small meatballs.

2. Heat the remaining olive oil over medium-high heat in a large nonstick pan. Add the meatballs. Cook for about 5 minutes, turning so that the meatballs brown on all sides. (Note that meatballs will be returned to the pan later; so they do not have to be cooked through yet, just browned. If the oil starts to smoke, reduce the heat.) Remove the meatballs to a plate.

3. Cook the sliced mushrooms in the same pan over medium-high heat for 8 to 12 minutes, until golden brown and all of their water has been released and evaporated.

4. Squeeze the lemon juice into the pan and deglaze it, scraping the bottom of the pan with a wooden spoon or spatula.

5. Meanwhile, in a small bowl, whisk together the flour and the stock, and add the mixture to the mushrooms in the pan. Return the meatballs to the pan as well, bring the stock mixture to a simmer, and cook until the meatballs are just cooked through and the sauce has thickened, about 2 minutes.

6. Remove the meatballs from the sauce, and place on a nice platter. Add the sour cream to the pan, stirring over low heat until well combined.

7. In a small saucepan, heat the jam separately until warmed.

8. Spoon the sauce over the meatballs. Top the meatballs with dollops of jam and sprinkle with the parsley. Serve with toothpicks.

Small Bites

CALORIES **197**

TOTAL FAT **9 G**

CHOLESTEROL **28 MG**

SATURATED FAT **2 G**

TOTAL CARBOHYDRATES **17 G**

FIBER **2 G**

SUGAR **3 G**

SODIUM **614 MG**

PROTEIN **14 G**

Smoked Salmon on Crostini

SERVES 5

PREPARATION TIME **5 MINUTES**
COOKING TIME **10 MINUTES**
TOTAL TIME **15 MINUTES**

These little sandwiches are a play on the bagel with everything and can be served any time of day as an hors d'oeuvre or eaten as a snack.

When it comes to choosing the type of salmon to use on the crostini, you have the option of smoked salmon, lox (salmon cured in brine), or gravlax (salmon cured in a rub of sugar, salt, and dill), each with its own particular flavor, and all great options.

1 pumpernickel baguette, sliced into thin crostini
Olive oil cooking spray
Fine-grained kosher salt, to taste
¼ cup nonfat sour cream
¼ cup nonfat cream cheese
2 tablespoons finely chopped dill
1 red onion, sliced thinly
10 to 12 slices smoked salmon, lox, or gravlax
¼ cup capers

1. Preheat the oven to 375 degrees F.

2. Spray the crostini with olive oil cooking spray on both sides, sprinkle with salt, and toast for 8 to 12 minutes or until crispy.

3. In a small bowl, combine the sour cream, cream cheese, and dill until well incorporated. Put the mixture in a blender to purée if necessary.

4. Smear the creamy dill spread on the pumpernickel slices.

5. Top each crostini with a thin slice of red onion, a slice of salmon, and some capers.

CALORIES **155**
TOTAL FAT **4 G**
CHOLESTEROL **20 MG**
SATURATED FAT **1 G**
TOTAL CARBOHYDRATES **14 G**

FIBER **1 G**
SUGAR **2 G**
SODIUM **294 MG**
PROTEIN **16 G**

CHAPTER FOUR

Snacks and Dips

Cool Ranch Dip

Crispy Sweet Potato Chips with
Pumpkin–White Bean Dip

Baked Potato Chips with French
Onion Dip

Green Goddess Dip with Crudités

Extra-Loaded Nachos Supreme

Garlic Hummus

Zesty, Herbed Marinated Olives

Perfect Parmesan Popcorn

Baked Tortilla Chips with Sweet
and Spicy Fruit Salsa

CHAPTER FOUR

Snacks and Dips

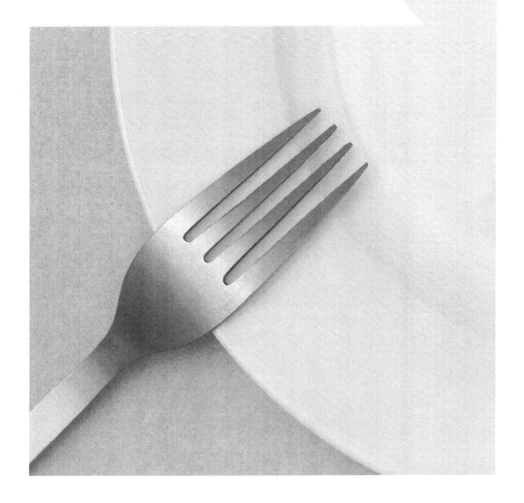

Cool Ranch Dip

PREPARATION TIME **10 MINUTES**
COOKING TIME **3 MINUTES**
TOTAL TIME **13 MINUTES**

This flavorful yogurt-based dip is ideal for serving along with crudités, chips, pretzels, breaded chicken tenders, or buffalo wings. Don't skimp on the spices, and buy a good-quality Greek yogurt to use as the base for the sauce.

1 cup nonfat Greek yogurt
½ cup nonfat sour cream or additional ½ cup nonfat Greek yogurt
⅓ cup buttermilk
2 tablespoons fresh lemon juice
½ teaspoon Dijon mustard
¼ teaspoon ground coriander
½ teaspoon garlic powder
3 tablespoons finely chopped chives
5 fresh basil leaves, finely chopped
½ teaspoon dried tarragon
½ teaspoon dried dill weed (optional)
Fine-grained kosher salt and freshly ground black pepper, to taste

1. In a medium bowl, whisk the yogurt, sour cream, buttermilk, lemon juice, Dijon mustard, coriander, and garlic powder together until well combined.

2. Whisk in the chives, basil, tarragon, and dill weed. Season with salt and pepper.

3. Store in an airtight container in the refrigerator for up to 4 days.

CALORIES **88**
TOTAL FAT **1 G**
CHOLESTEROL **7 MG**
SATURATED FAT **1 G**
TOTAL CARBOHYDRATES **14 G**

FIBER **3 G**
SUGAR **6 G**
SODIUM **115 MG**
PROTEIN **6 G**

Crisp Sweet Potato Chips with Pumpkin-White Bean Dip

SERVES 8

PREPARATION TIME **10 MINUTES**
COOKING TIME **15 TO 25 MINUTES**
TOTAL TIME **25 TO 30 MINUTES**

The best way to prepare these chips is to bake them in the oven with a convection setting, because the circulating dry air makes them extra crisp. A regular oven will also work, and you can use the microwave (as directed below). The only drawback to this is that you have to make the chips in small batches.

4 garlic cloves
2 tablespoons olive oil
1½ cups canned cannellini beans, rinsed and drained
1½ cups canned unsweetened pumpkin purée
Pinch of freshly grated nutmeg
Fine-grained kosher salt and freshly ground white pepper, to taste
5 medium sweet potatoes
Olive oil cooking spray, to coat

1. To prepare the dip, first caramelize the garlic. Smash the garlic cloves with the side of a knife, and remove the skins. Place the smashed garlic in a sauté pan, and add enough olive oil to just cover the garlic.

2. Cook over medium-high heat for 5 to 7 minutes. The garlic should brown and the oil should bubble. Remove the garlic immediately. Let the oil cool down, and reserve.

3. In a standing blender or with an immersion blender, purée the white beans with the pumpkin, smashed caramelized garlic, and the olive oil reserved from roasting the garlic. Add the nutmeg. Stir and season with salt and pepper. Set the dip aside for the flavors to meld while you prepare the chips.

4. Preheat the oven to 400 degrees F.

5. Wash and pat the sweet potatoes dry. Use a mandoline, set on a thin setting, to create very thin slices. (See "Caution: Using a Mandoline" on page 55.)

6. Put the slices in a large bowl, and spray with oil evenly to coat. Sprinkle the slices with salt.

7. Place the slices in a single, even layer on baking sheets covered with parchment paper (if you don't have parchment paper, just make sure the chips are well oiled). Bake the chips for 12 to 15 minutes, or until they begin to brown slightly.

8. Serve the dip with the chips, and enjoy!

To Make the Chips in a Microwave

After oiling and salting the chips, arrange as many as will fit in one layer on a microwave-safe plate that has a light coating of cooking spray. Microwave on high power for 1 to 2 minutes, checking after 1 minute. The plate should be removed with an oven mitt or folded dry towel, as it will be very hot to the touch. Continue microwaving in batches until all of the chips are crispy.

Caution: Using a Mandoline

Mandolines are notorious in restaurant kitchens for causing deep cuts on hands and fingers. Always exercise caution when using a mandoline. Make a few slices to get a flat side on the vegetable. If you use your hand, use only the palm of your hand on the vegetable and keep your fingers up. Use the guard to slice. When there is a nub of vegetable left and the guard no longer works or your hand is too close, save that end of the vegetable for another purpose, such as mashed sweet potatoes. Mandolines are extremely sharp! Your hand and fingers should never get close to the blade. Always keep your eyes on the mandoline and the vegetable when you are using it. Keep the blade sharp, so you do not have to press too hard on the vegetable. The mandoline is even more dangerous when the blade is dull.

CALORIES **186**

TOTAL FAT **5 G**

CHOLESTEROL **0 MG**

SATURATED FAT **1 G**

TOTAL CARBOHYDRATES **33 G**

FIBER **8 G**

SUGAR **7 G**

SODIUM **200 MG**

PROTEIN **5 G**

Baked Potato Chips with French Onion Dip

SERVES 5

PREPARATION TIME **20 MINUTES**
COOKING TIME **20 MINUTES**
TOTAL TIME **40 MINUTES**

Sure, you can buy potato chips anywhere, but have you ever tried making your own? You control how much salt you put in, what kind of oil you use, and most important, you'll really be able to taste the difference.

The best way to thinly slice the potatoes is to use a mandoline. You don't need an expensive metal French-style mandoline; a thin $20 plastic slicer would work just fine (see "Caution: Using a Mandoline" on page 55). Don't have a mandoline? Don't despair. Other alternatives include a super sharp chef's knife to shave thin slices from the potato (this can be tricky), a vegetable peeler (the resulting shape may be funny, but thin is the goal), or the blade attachment of a food processor.

5 medium Idaho potatoes
Olive oil cooking spray, to coat
1 teaspoon fine-grained kosher salt, plus more, to taste
2 tablespoons canola oil
2 large red onions, chopped
½ cup beef stock or water, divided
2 garlic cloves, minced
1 tablespoon fresh thyme
Freshly ground black pepper, to taste
1 tablespoon Worcestershire sauce
12 ounces plain nonfat Greek yogurt or nonfat sour cream
8 ounces nonfat cream cheese, at room temperature

1. Preheat the oven to 400 degrees F.

2. Use a mandoline, set to a thin setting, to create very thin slices.

3. Put the slices in a large bowl and spray with oil evenly to coat. Sprinkle with salt.

4. Arrange the slices in a single layer on baking sheets covered with parchment paper (if you don't have any parchment paper, that's fine, as long as the chips are well oiled).

5. Bake chips for about 12 to 15 minutes or until they begin to brown.

6. Meanwhile, heat the canola oil in a large skillet over high heat until hot and shimmering.

7. Add the onions and 1 tablespoon of the beef stock, and sprinkle with 1 teaspoon of kosher salt. Continue to let the onions sizzle.

8. Keep adding 1 tablespoon of the stock as it evaporates.

9. Continue cooking the onions, flipping them periodically, until they are brown and caramelized, but not burnt.

10. Add the minced garlic and fresh thyme, and cook for 30 seconds.

11. Season with pepper, add the Worcestershire sauce, stir, and remove from the heat.

12. In a blender or food processor, purée together the sour cream or yogurt and the cream cheese. Empty the mixture into a bowl, and add the onions and seasonings.

13. Season with more salt and pepper. Serve alongside the baked potato chips.

To Make the Chips in a Microwave

After oiling and salting the chips, arrange as many as will fit in one layer on a microwave-safe plate that has a light coating of cooking spray. Microwave on high power for 1 to 2 minutes, checking after 1 minute. The plate should be removed with an oven mitt or folded dry towel, as it will be very hot to the touch. Continue microwaving in batches until all of the chips are crispy.

CALORIES **173**

TOTAL FAT **7 G**

CHOLESTEROL **10 MG**

SATURATED FAT **1 G**

TOTAL CARBOHYDRATES **16 G**

FIBER **1 G**

SUGAR **10 G**

SODIUM **421 MG**

PROTEIN **12 G**

Green Goddess Dip with Crudités

SERVES 10

PREPARATION TIME **10 MINUTES**
COOKING TIME **15 MINUTES**
TOTAL TIME **25 MINUTES**

Crunchy veggies serve as the spoons for this heavenly, rich avocado-based dip. Try using celery stalks and cucumbers too, which you seed first, then fill the cavity with the dip.

You may be surprised to see anchovies in the ingredients. Even if you're not a fan, you might make an exception for the white Spanish anchovies called boquerones—*they aren't fishy because they're pickled in vinegar; they are flavorful and delicious. (Worcestershire sauce itself contains puréed anchovies for that mildly salty flavor that's hard to beat.)*

1 lemon, freshly squeezed
1 shallot or ¼ red onion, finely chopped
2 whole anchovy fillets
1 garlic clove, minced
1 tablespoon white wine vinegar
2 large avocados, peeled and pitted, pits reserved
½ cup nonfat sour cream or nonfat Greek yogurt
¼ cup chopped fresh parsley
3 tablespoons finely chopped fresh tarragon or ½ tablespoon
    dried tarragon
8 fresh basil leaves, finely chopped
½ cup extra-virgin olive oil
Fine-grained kosher salt and freshly ground black pepper, to taste
1 head broccoli florets
1 head cauliflower florets
5 carrots, peeled and cut into sticks
1 pint baby tomatoes
4 stalks celery, leaves and tough parts removed, cut into sticks
1 red or yellow bell pepper, cored, seeded, and cut into wide strips

1. To prepare the dip, combine the lemon juice, shallots, anchovies, garlic, and vinegar in a food processor or blender. Purée until all of the ingredients are well combined.

2. Add the avocado, sour cream, and the herbs. Purée until smooth, and then reduce the speed to low.

3. While the blender is running, gradually pour in the olive oil. Continue to blend until fully incorporated and creamy.

4. Put the dip into a bowl. Season with salt and pepper. Stir and push the pits into the dip. (They help to keep it bright green.)

5. Cover and place the dip in the refrigerator. It can be made up to 24 hours in advance and kept chilled.

6. To prepare the crudités, blanch the broccoli florets by submerging them in salted boiling water for about 5 minutes, or until just tender but still crisp and bright green.

7. Remove the broccoli from the boiling water, and submerge it in ice-cold water. Let the broccoli sit to cool for 1 minute at most, then drain.

8. Place the broccoli on a platter and chill.

9. Next, blanch the cauliflower florets until slightly tender and bright white. Repeat the process of submerging it in ice-cold water to cool, and then drain and chill.

10. Serve the rest of the vegetables as is, placed on the serving tray or platter with the cauliflower and the broccoli, with the dip on the side.

CALORIES **233**

TOTAL FAT **18 G**

CHOLESTEROL **5 MG**

SATURATED FAT **3 G**

TOTAL CARBOHYDRATES **16 G**

FIBER **6 G**

SUGAR **5 G**

SODIUM **258 MG**

PROTEIN **5 G**

Extra-Loaded Nachos Supreme

SERVES 10

PREPARATION TIME **15 MINUTES**
COOKING TIME **15 MINUTES**
TOTAL TIME **30 MINUTES**

Sometimes when watching the game or a romantic comedy, a snack that has it all—crunchy, creamy, salty, and spicy—is the best. In these super-loaded nachos, layers of bean dip, guacamole, fresh "pico de gallo" salsa, and cheese sauce top crisp baked corn tortilla chips.

For the next game party or poker game, when you are having ten guests or so, make this party-size recipe. It's easy to reduce the recipe for fewer eaters.

3 avocados, peeled and pitted

Juice of 2 limes, divided

Fine-grained kosher salt, to taste

1 can black beans, rinsed and drained

1 chipotle from a can of chipotles in adobo sauce, minced, or
      1 tablespoon hot sauce

2 tablespoons water

4 ripe beefsteak or hothouse tomatoes or 5 plum (Italian Roma)
      tomatoes, finely chopped

1 jalapeño, chopped finely

½ cup chopped cilantro or parsley leaves

6 sliced scallions (optional)

15 medium-size corn tortillas (or 20 small-size), sliced into
      8 (or more) triangle-shaped pieces

Olive oil cooking spray

1 tablespoon olive oil

1 tablespoon all-purpose flour

1 cup 1 percent milk

Pinch of grated nutmeg

½ cup reduced-fat sharp cheddar cheese

Freshly ground white pepper, to taste

1. Make the guacamole by mashing the avocados with half the lime juice and a sprinkle of salt. Set aside.

2. To prepare the bean dip, combine the beans, chipotle or hot sauce, and water in a blender and purée on high until smooth. Add more water while blending if necessary to achieve desired consistency. Season with salt. Set aside.

3. To prepare the salsa, combine the tomatoes, remaining lime juice, jalapeño, cilantro, and scallions, if using. Season with salt. Set aside.

4. To bake the chips, preheat the oven to 375 degrees F. Coat the chips with the cooking spray, sprinkle with salt, and place on baking sheets covered with parchment paper (you can skip the parchment paper as long as the chips are well oiled). Bake for 12 minutes or until crispy and golden.

5. Meanwhile, prepare the cheese sauce. In a saucepan, over medium-high heat, whisk the olive oil and flour constantly for 3 to 5 minutes, until it reaches a golden hue and has a nutty fragrance. (Do not stop whisking or the roux will burn.)

6. Reduce the heat to medium, and slowly drizzle in the milk, whisking briskly the whole time. The sauce will become the consistency of very thick cream. The nutmeg can be grated directly into the sauce or measured out. Use the side of a box grater, a nutmeg or spice grater, or a microplane. If you're grating the nutmeg directly into the sauce, 1 or 2 scrapes equals a pinch.

7. Remove the milk mixture from the heat, and whisk in the grated cheddar. Season with salt and pepper.

8. To assemble the nachos, place the tortilla chips on a platter, spoon on the bean dip, add the guacamole, the salsa, and drizzle the cheese sauce on top.

Snacks and Dips

CALORIES **303**

TOTAL FAT **16 G**

CHOLESTEROL **8 MG**

SATURATED FAT **3 G**

TOTAL CARBOHYDRATES **36 G**

FIBER **10 G**

SUGAR **2 G**

SODIUM **986 MG**

PROTEIN **9 G**

Garlic Hummus

SERVES 8

PREPARATION TIME **5 MINUTES**
COOKING TIME **0 MINUTES**
TOTAL TIME **5 MINUTES**

Dip crudités, baked tortilla chips (see page 66), or pita chips in this simple, garlicky hummus. Tahini, or sesame seed paste, is what gives hummus its traditional, characteristic flavor. Nonetheless, the tahini paste can be omitted if you don't have any on hand.

1 (15- to 16-ounce) can chickpeas, rinsed and drained
Juice of 1 lemon
2 garlic cloves, minced
1 teaspoon ground cumin
1 tablespoon tahini paste
1½ teaspoons paprika
¼ cup water
2 tablespoons extra-virgin olive oil, divided
Fine-grained kosher salt and freshly ground black pepper, to taste
¼ cup finely chopped parsley, for garnish
4 whole-wheat pita breads, cut in wedges

1. Purée the chickpeas, lemon juice, garlic, cumin, tahini, paprika, water, and 1 tablespoon of the olive oil in a blender or food processor on high speed until the hummus is very creamy.

2. Pour the hummus into a mixing bowl. Season with salt and pepper, and stir.

3. To serve, place the hummus in a serving bowl, drizzle the top with the remaining olive oil, and sprinkle with the parsley to garnish.

4. Serve with the pita bread.

CALORIES **142**
TOTAL FAT **5 G**
CHOLESTEROL **0 MG**
SATURATED FAT **1 G**
TOTAL CARBOHYDRATES **20G**

FIBER **3 G**
SUGAR **0 G**
SODIUM **202 MG**
PROTEIN **4G**

Zesty, Herbed Marinated Olives

SERVES 16

PREPARATION TIME **5 MINUTES**
COOKING TIME **2 HOURS (SIMMERING)**
TOTAL TIME **2 HOURS 5 MINUTES**

This is a great recipe to make well ahead of time, because the olives can be refrigerated in cooking marinade for up to two weeks. When the olives are gone, strain the marinade, and use the remaining oil as a dressing.

1 cup green olives, drained (don't rinse)
1 cup kalamata olives, drained (don't rinse)
1 cup olive oil
½ cup red wine vinegar
3 whole garlic cloves, peeled
3 rosemary sprigs
Zest of 1 orange
Zest of 1 lemon
1 bay leaf
1 tablespoon black peppercorns (optional)
1 tablespoon whole coriander seeds (optional)

1. Put all ingredients in a medium pot, and let simmer over medium-low heat for 2 hours.

2. Remove from the heat and let cool.

3. Refrigerate before serving.

Perfect Parmesan Popcorn

SERVES 6

PREPARATION TIME **3 MINUTES**
COOKING TIME **10 MINUTES**
TOTAL TIME **13 MINUTES**

Grating fresh Parmesan cheese into this popcorn gives it unbeatable flavor, but the best way to achieve maximum taste is to make the popcorn on the stove top with a touch of oil. You can also save calories by air-popping popcorn, or save time by purchasing natural microwavable popcorn in the bag. By using the Parmesan cheese, little if any salt will be needed.

3 tablespoons canola oil
⅓ cup popcorn kernels
½ cup finely grated Parmesan cheese
Fine-grained kosher salt and freshly ground black pepper, to taste

1. In a heavy-bottomed pot, heat the oil over medium heat until shimmering but not smoky. (If the oil smokes, turn down the heat.)

2. To test if the oil is hot enough, place 3 popcorn kernels into the pan. As soon as they pop, the oil is hot enough; add more popcorn until they form an even layer on the bottom of the pan.

3. Cover the pot, shake it to coat the kernels with oil (take care not to spill the oil), and remove from heat for 30 seconds.

4. Put the pot back over medium heat. The popcorn should begin popping right away. Move the pot back and forth on the stove top to shake gently.

5. Let the lid be slightly loose so that some steam can escape.

6. When the popping slows to about 3 seconds between pops, remove the pot from the heat and dump the popcorn into a bowl, discarding any remaining kernels.

7. Add the Parmesan cheese, and season with salt and pepper.

CALORIES **100**

TOTAL FAT **10 G**

CHOLESTEROL **7 MG**

SATURATED FAT **2 G**

TOTAL CARBOHYDRATES **1 G**

FIBER **0 G**

SUGAR **0 G**

SODIUM **128 MG**

PROTEIN **3 G**

Baked Tortilla Chips with Sweet and Spicy Fruit Salsa

SERVES 8

PREPARATION TIME **5 MINUTES**
COOKING TIME **12 TO 15 MINUTES (TO BAKE TORTILLA CHIPS)**
TOTAL TIME **17 TO 20 MINUTES**

In this recipe, the fruity salsa is served with baked tortilla chips, but you can also serve it as a sauce over fish, pork, or chicken for a pop of sweet, fresh flavor.

1 cup finely chopped peaches
2 cups finely chopped strawberries
½ cup chopped cherries or chopped plums or pomegranate seeds
1 jalapeño, stemmed, seeded, and finely chopped
1 garlic clove, finely minced
Juice of 1 medium orange
½ cup coarsely chopped fresh cilantro, parsley, mint, or basil leaves
Fine-grained kosher salt, to taste
10 medium to large soft corn tortillas, cut into 8 (or more) wedges
Olive oil cooking spray or 1 teaspoon olive oil

1. Mix together the fruit, jalapeño, garlic, orange juice, and herbs in a medium bowl.

2. Season with salt and place in a serving bowl.

3. Let the flavors meld while you make the baking chips. (Salsa can be stored in the refrigerator overnight.)

4. Preheat the oven to 375 degrees F.

5. Coat the chips with the cooking spray, season with salt, and place on baking sheets covered with parchment paper (you can skip the parchment paper as long as the chips are well oiled).

6. Bake the chips for 12 minutes, or until crispy and golden.

7. Serve the chips in a platter or bowl alongside the salsa.

CALORIES **52**

TOTAL FAT **1 G**

CHOLESTEROL **0 MG**

SATURATED FAT **0 G**

TOTAL CARBOHYDRATES **11 G**

FIBER **2 G**

SUGAR **6 G**

SODIUM **195 MG**

PROTEIN **1 G**

Traditional Salads

Traditional Salads

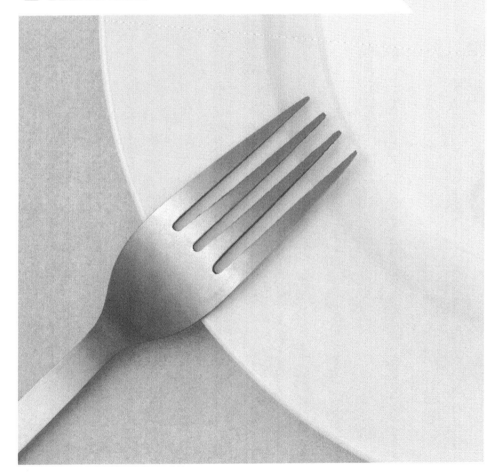

Mozzarella, Basil, and Tomato Caprese Salad

SERVES 8

PREPARATION TIME **10 MINUTES**
COOKING TIME **0 MINUTES**
TOTAL TIME **10 MINUTES**

This salad calls for fresh mozzarella mixed with tomatoes and basil. Often it's sprinkled with olive oil and balsamic vinegar. Here, the recipe calls for fresh lemon juice and olive oil, and the caprese ingredients are tossed with arugula or mixed spring greens to get a full green salad with a bright, fresh flavor. (If you find arugula's peppery taste too bitter, use spring greens.)

1 package prewashed baby arugula or mixed spring greens
25 fresh basil leaves
1 (8-ounce) package low-fat mozzarella
2 tomatoes cut into wedges
¼ cup extra-virgin olive oil
juice of 1 lemon
Fine-grained kosher salt and freshly ground pepper, to taste

1. Place the arugula or greens in a large salad bowl. Tear up the basil leaves and add to the salad. Chop the mozzarella into bite-size pieces, and add them to the salad, along with the tomatoes.

2. Drizzle the salad with the olive oil and lemon juice, and season with salt and pepper. Toss well to combine, and add more olive oil, lemon juice, or salt and pepper if needed.

CALORIES **157**
TOTAL FAT **13 G**
CHOLESTEROL **18 MG**
SATURATED FAT **4 G**
TOTAL CARBOHYDRATES **3 G**

FIBER **1 G**
SUGAR **1 G**
SODIUM **250 MG**
PROTEIN **7 G**

Curry Apple Potato Salad

PREPARATION TIME **45 MINUTES (INCLUDING 30 MINUTES COOLING TIME)**
COOKING TIME **25 MINUTES (INCLUDING BOILING WATER)**
TOTAL TIME **1 HOUR 10 MINUTES (INCLUDING 30 MINUTES COOLING TIME)**

Mild yellow curry adds warmth to this potato salad, and apples add crunch and sweetness. You can serve this salad with some grilled bratwurst for an interesting cookout meal.

3 pounds potatoes, scrubbed clean and chopped into
    bite-size pieces
1 tablespoon fine-grained kosher salt, plus more, to taste
½ cup nonfat mayonnaise
¾ cup nonfat sour cream or nonfat Greek yogurt
2 tablespoons yellow curry powder
½ cup raisins or dried cranberries (or mix of both)
2 Granny Smith apples
2 tablespoons fresh lemon juice
2 stalks celery, finely chopped
1 medium red onion, finely chopped

1. Put the potatoes and 1 tablespoon of salt in a pot of cold water. Bring the water to a boil, and allow the potatoes to cook for about 10 minutes more, or until the potatoes are slightly tender when pierced with a fork or the tip of a knife.

2. Strain the potatoes through a colander.

3. Whisk together the mayonnaise, sour cream or yogurt, and curry powder to make the dressing.

4. Season with salt, then cover and place in the refrigerator.

5. Spread the potatoes in a single layer on a platter or baking sheet lined with parchment or wax paper, and put them in the refrigerator to cool for about 30 minutes. (Note that the potatoes do not have to become totally cold.)

6. In the meantime, plump the raisins or cranberries in hot water, covering the fruit by ½ inch, and allow to sit for 20 minutes.

7. Peel, core, and dice the apples. Toss in lemon juice to coat.

8. Remove the cooled potatoes from the refrigerator and place them in a large bowl.

9. Fold in the refrigerated dressing. Add the apples, celery, and onion.

10. Drain the plumped raisins or cranberries, and add them to the potato salad.

11. Toss well, cover, and refrigerate for a few hours to allow the flavors to blend.

12. Serve cold or at room temperature.

CALORIES **206**

TOTAL FAT **8 G**

CHOLESTEROL **1 MG**

SATURATED FAT **1 G**

TOTAL CARBOHYDRATES **32 G**

FIBER **4 G**

SUGAR **4 G**

SODIUM **150 MG**

PROTEIN **3 G**

Mex-Asian Coleslaw

SERVES 12

PREPARATION TIME **20 MINUTES**
COOKING TIME **0 MINUTES**
TOTAL TIME **20 MINUTES**

A little spice, a little crunch, a creamy dressing with some ginger juice and toasted sesame seeds—this new take on coleslaw is jam-packed with flavor. What a bright and refreshing side salad!

As with any coleslaw, this dish is best served after it has chilled in the refrigerator for a few hours or overnight, so that the flavors meld.

1 large piece fresh gingerroot
2 tablespoons sesame seeds
1 head Napa or green cabbage, finely shredded
2 large carrots, peeled and shredded
Juice of 2 limes, divided
¾ cup nonfat mayonnaise
¼ cup nonfat sour cream or nonfat Greek yogurt
¼ cup thinly sliced scallions or red onion
2 Granny Smith, McIntosh, or Golden Delicious Apples, diced
½ teaspoon ground cumin
⅛ teaspoon cayenne pepper
¼ cup chopped fresh cilantro or parsley
Fine-grained kosher salt, to taste

1. Start by juicing the ginger: wash the gingerroot; grate it on the fine side of a box grater, with a microplane, or with a ginger grater; and then squeeze the gingerroot through a cheesecloth. You need 2 tablespoons of ginger juice for the salad.

2. Toast the sesame seeds by placing them in a sauté pan over low heat for 4 minutes, stirring constantly until they turn golden and release a nutty fragrance.

3. In a large bowl, mix together the cabbage, carrots, and half of the lime juice.

4. In a separate bowl, mix together the mayonnaise, sour cream or Greek yogurt, scallions or onion, apples, ginger juice, the rest of the lime juice, cumin, and cayenne pepper to make the dressing.

5. Add the dressing to the cabbage and stir in to combine thoroughly.

6. Add the cilantro or parsley, and season with salt, as desired.

CALORIES **162**

TOTAL FAT **13 G**

CHOLESTEROL **1 MG**

SATURATED FAT **2 G**

TOTAL CARBOHYDRATES **11 G**

FIBER **3 G**

SUGAR **6 G**

SODIUM **170 MG**

PROTEIN **2 G**

Cobb Salad

PREPARATION TIME **10 MINUTES**

COOKING TIME **10 MINUTES (ADD TIME IF CHICKEN AND EGGS ARE NOT PRECOOKED)**

TOTAL TIME **20 MINUTES**

Protein-packed and filling, this traditional Cobb salad is a meal on its own. The dressing is light and simple, so it won't overwhelm the salad. Don't forget that a traditional Cobb salad is served with the ingredients on top of the greens, rather than tossed to combine.

2 avocados, peeled, pitted, and chopped into bite-size pieces

2 tablespoons fresh lemon juice, plus more for seasoning

6 slices of turkey bacon, crumbled

1 tablespoon Dijon mustard

1 teaspoon granulated sucralose (optional)

½ cup extra-virgin olive oil

Fine-grained kosher salt and freshly ground pepper, to taste

1 head romaine lettuce

½ cup reduced-fat blue cheese crumbles

2 hard-boiled eggs, sliced

1 cooked chicken breast (skin removed), chopped

1. Toss the chopped avocado in lemon juice so it will not brown. Set aside.

2. Cook the bacon on both sides over medium heat in a sauté pan or skillet, for about 5 minutes on each side, or until crisp.

3. Line a plate with paper towels, remove each strip of bacon with a fork or tongs, and lay on the plate. Cover with a layer of paper towels to remove extra grease.

4. In a small bowl, whisk together the 2 tablespoons lemon juice, mustard, and sucralose, if using.

5. Gradually add the oil in a steady and slow drizzle while whisking. Keep whisking until the dressing appears creamy, and the oil and lemon juice seem combined.

6. Season with salt and pepper.

7. Coarsely chop the romaine lettuce. Combine the romaine lettuce and the dressing in a large bowl, and toss well to combine.

8. When ready to serve, place the salad in individual salad bowls or a large serving platter.

9. Top the salad with the crumbled blue cheese, bacon, hard-boiled egg slices, chicken, and avocado.

CALORIES **379**

TOTAL FAT **35 G**

CHOLESTEROL **70 MG**

SATURATED FAT **8 G**

TOTAL CARBOHYDRATES **9 G**

FIBER **5 G**

SUGAR **2 G**

SODIUM **200 MG**

PROTEIN **11 G**

Tuna Macaroni Salad

SERVES 10

PREPARATION TIME **15 MINUTES**
COOKING TIME **20 MINUTES (INCLUDING BOILING WATER)**
TOTAL TIME **35 MINUTES**

This is an updated version of a traditional macaroni salad that includes both regular and whole-wheat pasta, making for an interesting texture and visual appeal. If you're out of macaroni, penne or farfalle are also good options.

1 cup elbow macaroni
1 cup whole-wheat elbow macaroni
½ cup nonfat mayonnaise
¾ teaspoon Dijon mustard
1½ teaspoons sucralose
1½ tablespoons white vinegar
¼ cup nonfat Greek yogurt or nonfat sour cream
Fine-grained kosher salt and freshly ground black pepper, to taste
2 (8-ounce) cans tuna in water (albacore or other)
2 stalks celery, finely chopped
1 red onion, finely chopped
2 tablespoons finely chopped parsley
½ teaspoon paprika

1. Cook the macaroni according to the package directions. When done, rinse with cool water and drain completely.

2. In a small bowl, whisk together the mayonnaise, mustard, sucralose, vinegar, yogurt or sour cream, and season with salt and pepper to make the dressing.

3. Combine the tuna, celery, red onion, parsley, and paprika in a large bowl.

4. Stir the macaroni into the vegetables; then add the dressing, and stir well. Season with more salt and pepper, if needed.

5. The pasta salad will taste best if you let it stand for a few hours in the refrigerator, and it can be stored for up to 3 days.

CALORIES **227**
TOTAL FAT **10 G**
CHOLESTEROL **14 MG**
SATURATED FAT **2 G**
TOTAL CARBOHYDRATES **18 G**

FIBER **1 G**
SUGAR **2 G**
SODIUM **201 MG**
PROTEIN **15 G**

Waldorf Salad

SERVES 8

PREPARATION TIME **15 MINUTES**
COOKING TIME **0 MINUTES (IF NUTS ARE TOASTED IN ADVANCE)**
TOTAL TIME **15 MINUTES**

This is a refreshing crunchy salad with walnuts, celery, and crisp apples. The juiciness of the grapes is nice, too! (But if you don't have grapes on hand, substitute ¼ cup of raisins.)

It is better to toast nuts whole and then chop later—there's less mess and they retain more flavor.

1 apple, peeled, cored, and chopped
2 tablespoons fresh lemon juice, divided
2 tablespoons nonfat mayonnaise
2 tablespoons nonfat Greek yogurt
Fine-grained kosher salt and freshly ground black pepper
1 head romaine lettuce or ½ head romaine lettuce plus ½ head frisée,
     torn or chopped into bite-size pieces
½ cup thinly sliced celery
½ cup sliced red seedless grapes
½ cup walnuts, toasted and chopped

1. Toss chopped apples in half of the lemon juice to prevent browning. Set aside.

2. In a small bowl, whisk together the mayonnaise, yogurt, and the rest of the lemon juice to make the dressing.

3. Season with salt and pepper.

4. In a large bowl, toss together the lettuce, apples in lemon juice, celery, grapes, and walnuts.

5. Add the dressing to the bowl and toss, fully incorporating it into the salad.

CALORIES **142**
TOTAL FAT **12 G**
CHOLESTEROL **0 MG**
SATURATED FAT **1 G**
TOTAL CARBOHYDRATES **8 G**

FIBER **3 G**
SUGAR **4 G**
SODIUM **271 MG**
PROTEIN **3 G**

Caesar Salad

SERVES 6

PREPARATION TIME **10 MINUTES**
COOKING TIME **10 MINUTES (FOR THE CROUTONS)**
TOTAL TIME **20 MINUTES**

This recipe is the traditional version of a wonderful classic, but made with mayonnaise rather than the raw egg and oil. This dish can be turned into an entrée by adding some grilled or roasted chicken breast, or grilled shrimp or salmon (but remember that the overall nutritional content of your meal would be changed).

1 whole-wheat, sourdough, or pumpernickel baguette, chopped (stale preferred)
Olive oil
Fine-grained kosher salt and freshly ground black pepper, to taste
2 cups nonfat mayonnaise
½ cup nonfat sour cream or nonfat Greek yogurt
1 tablespoon Dijon mustard
2 large garlic cloves, minced
8 anchovies (optional)
1 tablespoon Worcestershire sauce
Juice of 3 to 4 lemons
½ cup freshly grated Parmesan cheese
Dash of Tabasco sauce (optional)
1 large head romaine lettuce
1 pint cherry tomatoes, halved (optional)

1. Preheat the oven to 400 degrees F.

2. To make the croutons, drizzle the bread with plenty of olive oil, season with salt and pepper, and place the bread pieces in a single layer on a baking sheet lined with parchment paper (if you don't have parchment paper, just make sure your bread is well oiled).

3. Bake for 8 to 10 minutes until the croutons are golden and crisp.

4. Meanwhile, prepare the dressing. Blend the mayonnaise, sour cream or yogurt, mustard, garlic, anchovies, Worcestershire sauce, and lemon juice in a food processor or blender until well combined. Add the Parmesan cheese, and blend or pulse for 3 seconds, just until combined. Use a rubber spatula to empty the dressing into a small bowl. Season with salt and pepper. Stir in a dash of hot sauce, if using.

5. In a large bowl, combine the lettuce and cherry tomatoes, if using. Then add the dressing, hand-tossing to coat.

6. Divide the lettuce among 6 plates, and top with the homemade croutons.

CALORIES **130**

TOTAL FAT **6 G**

CHOLESTEROL **32 MG**

SATURATED FAT **2 G**

TOTAL CARBOHYDRATES **7 G**

FIBER **1 G**

SUGAR **3 G**

SODIUM **197 MG**

PROTEIN **14 G**

Traditional Salads

Crab Louis Salad

SERVES 6

PREPARATION TIME **15 MINUTES**
COOKING TIME **0 MINUTES**
TOTAL TIME **15 MINUTES**

This West Coast salad is popular from Seattle to San Francisco and is served with tomato wedges, hard-boiled eggs, and pink Louis dressing. Dungeness crab is the signature San Francisco ingredient.

½ cup nonfat mayonnaise
¼ cup no-sugar-added cocktail sauce
2 scallions, finely chopped
1 pound lump crabmeat
3 stalks celery, chopped
Fine-grained kosher salt and freshly ground black pepper
1 package (8 ounces) mesclun or spring greens
2 hard-boiled eggs, cut into wedges
1 beefsteak tomato, cut into wedges

1. In a medium bowl, combine the mayonnaise, cocktail sauce, and scallions to make the dressing. Set aside half in the refrigerator.

2. To the rest, stir in the crabmeat and celery until combined. Season with salt and pepper. Cover and refrigerate until ready to use.

3. When ready to serve, toss the salad greens with the reserved dressing, portion out on separate plates or salad bowls, and top each with the crab-meat mixture, eggs, and tomato.

CALORIES **228**
TOTAL FAT **2 G**
CHOLESTEROL **86 MG**
SATURATED FAT **1 G**
TOTAL CARBOHYDRATES **36 G**

FIBER **1 G**
SUGAR **34 G**
SODIUM **181 MG**
PROTEIN **17 G**

Spinach Salad

SERVES 8

PREPARATION TIME **15 MINUTES**
COOKING TIME **10 MINUTES**
TOTAL TIME **25 MINUTES**

This version of spinach salad is highly nutritious. Choose between walnuts or lean turkey bacon crumbles for crunch and protein, and add a touch of sweet with cranberries or raisins. The simple-to-make but rich, blue cheese dressing will have guests or family raving.

1 cup button mushrooms, sliced
½ tablespoon olive oil
½ cup nonfat mayonnaise
¼ nonfat sour cream or nonfat Greek yogurt
½ cup reduced-fat blue cheese crumbles
Fine-grained kosher salt and freshly ground black pepper, to taste
1 (10-ounce) package prewashed baby spinach
½ cup thinly sliced red onion or shallots
½ cup dried cranberries or raisins
5 strips lean turkey bacon, precooked and crumbled, or ½ cup
    walnuts, toasted
2 hard-boiled eggs, sliced (optional)

1. Place the mushrooms in olive oil in a sauté pan over medium heat, and cook until the mushrooms have lost much of their water and it has evaporated, or for about 8 minutes. Mushrooms should be golden and fragrant.

2. In a small bowl, whisk together the mayonnaise, sour cream or yogurt, and blue cheese crumbles, and season with salt and pepper to make the dressing.

3. In a large bowl, combine the mushrooms, spinach, onion or shallots, cranberries or raisins, and bacon or walnuts, and coat with the dressing. (Any remaining dressing can be stored in the refrigerator in an airtight container for up to 2 weeks.)

4. When ready to serve, garnish with eggs, if using.

CALORIES **159**
TOTAL FAT **12 G**
CHOLESTEROL **58 MG**
SATURATED FAT **4 G**
TOTAL CARBOHYDRATES **8 G**

FIBER **1 G**
SUGAR **6 G**
SODIUM **169 MG**
PROTEIN **6 G**

Ambrosia Fruit Salad

SERVES 8 TO 10

PREPARATION TIME **35 MINUTES**
COOKING TIME **6 MINUTES**
TOTAL TIME **41 MINUTES**

This is a popular fruit salad to serve at Thanksgiving or as a small treat for guests on other occasions: it's chewy, crunchy, sweet, and creamy, without the oily imitation whipped cream that may have given this salad a bad reputation. It's easy to make real whipped cream with nonfat evaporated milk, as shown here.

½ cup raisins or dried cranberries
½ cup whole walnuts
2 apples (preferably Granny Smith or similar)
2 tablespoons fresh lemon juice
2 (12-ounce) cans nonfat evaporated milk, chilled overnight
1 teaspoon pure vanilla extract
1 cup seedless red or green grapes, halved
2 peaches or nectarines, peeled, pitted, and chopped
½ pineapple, chopped (optional)
2 bananas, sliced

1. Plump the raisins or cranberries by covering them with hot water and soaking them for 20 minutes until fattened and juicy. Discard the water.

2. Roast the walnuts in a skillet over medium-low heat for about 6 minutes until golden and fragrant, stirring often. Remove from the heat, and allow to cool on a plate. After 5 to 10 minutes, coarsely chop the walnuts and set aside.

3. Meanwhile, peel, core, and chop the apples; place them in a small bowl; and toss with the lemon juice to prevent browning and add flavor. Set aside.

4. In the bowl of a standing mixer, using the whisk attachment, or in a bowl with an electric beater, whisk the evaporated milk and vanilla until stiff peaks form.

5. In a large bowl combine all of the fruit, plumped raisins or cranberries, and roasted walnuts, and fold in the whipped cream. Serve immediately.

CALORIES **139**

TOTAL FAT **4 G**

CHOLESTEROL **0 MG**

SATURATED FAT **0 G**

TOTAL CARBOHYDRATES **18 G**

FIBER **3 G**

SUGAR **11 G**

SODIUM **2 MG**

PROTEIN **3 G**

Zesty Black Bean and Corn Salad

SERVES 8 TO 10

PREPARATION TIME **15 MINUTES**
COOKING TIME **0 MINUTES**
TOTAL TIME **15 MINUTES**

Talk about a fiesta on a plate. There is so much flavor bursting from this colorful protein-packed salad that it will quickly become a favorite. And if you have leftovers, you can serve them as a bean and corn salsa with tortilla chips.

¼ cup extra-virgin olive oil
2 teaspoons ground cumin
2 garlic cloves, minced
⅛ teaspoon cayenne pepper
2 tablespoons fresh lime juice
Fine-grained kosher salt, to taste
2 cups canned black beans, rinsed and drained
1 red bell pepper, cored, seeded, and chopped
½ cup sliced scallions
2 cups corn kernels, fresh or thawed
1 jalapeño, seeded and finely chopped (optional)
½ cup finely chopped cilantro or parsley
1 avocado, peeled, pitted, and chopped
2 plum tomatoes or 1 ripe medium tomato, chopped

1. In a large bowl, whisk together the oil, cumin, garlic, cayenne pepper, and lime juice. Season with salt. (It's okay if the oil and juice do not blend together in the bowl. This is not supposed to be a creamy dressing.)

2. Now add the rest of the ingredients. Toss well to coat with the dressing. Taste and add more salt, if needed.

CALORIES **160**
TOTAL FAT **4 G**
CHOLESTEROL **0 MG**
SATURATED FAT **0 G**
TOTAL CARBOHYDRATES **14 G**

FIBER **6 G**
SUGAR **1 G**
SODIUM **150 MG**
PROTEIN **5 G**

Ten Classic Sandwiches

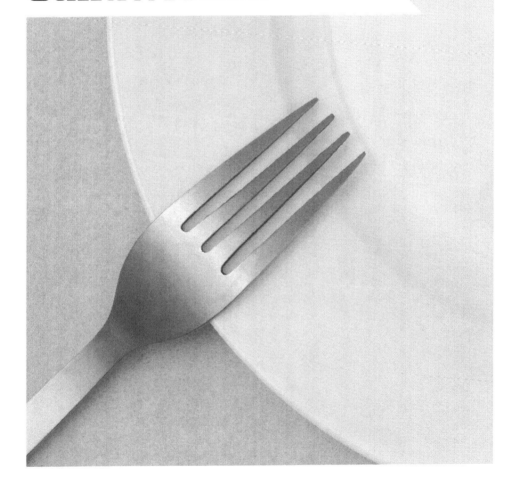

Ten Classic
Sandwiches

Open-Faced Reuben

SERVES 6

PREPARATION TIME **10 MINUTES**
COOKING TIME **10 MINUTES**
TOTAL TIME **20 MINUTES**

Open-faced sandwiches are great because only half of the bread is needed, thus cutting carbohydrates! If lean corned beef is unavailable, regular may be purchased, but keep in mind that the fat and sugar content of your sandwich will be affected.

Either Russian or Thousand Island dressing can be used. Both are a zingy combination of mayonnaise and ketchup, the difference being that Thousand Island contains pickled relish. Drain the sauerkraut well so that your sandwich doesn't get soggy before you're ready to enjoy it.

6 slices rye pumpernickel bread
2 tablespoons unsalted butter or olive oil
Fine-grained kosher salt, to taste
½ cup low-calorie Thousand Island or Russian dressing, divided
12 slices lean corned beef or pastrami or turkey pastrami
1 cup sauerkraut, well drained
6 slices reduced-fat Swiss cheese

1. Preheat the oven to 375 degrees F.

2. Lightly butter or coat one side of the bread slices with olive oil, sprinkle a small amount of salt evenly on each, and place the bread, buttered-side down, on a nonstick or parchment-lined baking sheet.

3. Spread the top of each bread slice with some of the dressing (reserving more for later), 2 slices of meat, one-sixth of the sauerkraut, and a slice of cheese.

4. Bake for about 10 minutes until golden brown on top and crisp on the bottom. Drizzle with the remaining dressing and serve.

CALORIES **343**
TOTAL FAT **6 G**
CHOLESTEROL **10 MG**
SATURATED FAT **1 G**
TOTAL CARBOHYDRATES **15 G**

FIBER **2 G**
SUGAR **4 G**
SODIUM **205 MG**
PROTEIN **21 G**

Chicago-Style Hot Dog

SERVES 6

PREPARATION TIME **10 MINUTES**
COOKING TIME **25 MINUTES**
TOTAL TIME **35 MINUTES**

The Midwestern metropolis boasts a hot dog that they say was "dragged through the garden," because there are so many vegetable toppings. Instead of ketchup, stick to tomato wedges—you don't need all that extra sugar.

6 reduced-fat beef, chicken, or turkey hot dogs
6 whole-wheat hot dog buns
1 tablespoon poppy seeds (optional)
6 dill pickle spears
¼ cup yellow mustard
¼ cup sweet green pickle relish
1 medium white onion, chopped
3 tomatoes, cut into wedges
12 banana peppers, Italian hot peppers, or "sport" peppers, seeded and chopped
1 teaspoon celery salt

1. You can either boil or grill the hot dogs. To boil, bring a medium pot of water to a boil over high heat.

2. Reduce heat to low, place the hot dogs in the simmering water, and cook for about 5 minutes until plumped and red.

3. Remove the hot dogs from the water with tongs, and set aside on a covered plate.

4. Alternately, grill the hot dogs over medium heat or flame until charred on all sides, or for about 5 minutes for a Chicago-style "char-dog."

5. Buns can be steamed by placing them in the microwave covered with a damp towel and cooking for 30 seconds, or by inserting a steamer basket into the pot of hot dog water (you may need to empty most of the water for this—water should not touch the basket). Cover the pot and steamer basket, and allow to sit off the heat for 1 minute. Remove the buns.

6. If using poppy seeds, spread them on a plate and press the steamed hot dog buns into the seeds so that some stick on each bun.

7. Place one pickle spear in each bun. Place a hot dog on top.

8. Now add the toppings: yellow mustard, sweet green pickle relish, onion, tomato wedges, and peppers. Sprinkle the dogs with some celery salt. Serve immediately.

CALORIES **325**

TOTAL FAT **5 G**

CHOLESTEROL **161 MG**

SATURATED FAT **1 G**

TOTAL CARBOHYDRATES **26 G**

FIBER **6 G**

SUGAR **10 G**

SODIUM **250 MG**

PROTEIN **10 G**

Monte Cristo Sandwich

SERVES 6 (½ SANDWICH PER SERVING)

PREPARATION TIME **20 MINUTES**
COOKING TIME **5 MINUTES**
TOTAL TIME **25 MINUTES**

This egg-dipped sandwich takes a simple ham and cheese to the next level. You don't need to visit a French bistro to enjoy this decadent dish. If you don't have any Gouda, Muenster cheese is a good substitute.

6 slices whole-wheat or sourdough bread
2 tablespoons nonfat mayonnaise
Fine-grained kosher salt, to taste
12 slices deli or home-roasted and thinly sliced turkey
3 slices low-fat Gouda
3 large eggs, beaten, or ¾ cup egg substitute
¼ cup milk
2 tablespoons olive oil (not extra-virgin)
1 tablespoon unsalted butter
6 tablespoons no-sugar-added cranberry chutney or
    no-sugar-added lingonberry, blackberry, or seedless
    raspberry jam

1. Spread the bread slices with a light layer of mayonnaise. Sprinkle with a small amount of salt. On the bottom piece of bread, put 2 slices of turkey and 1 slice of the cheese; make 3. Top each with a slice of bread to make 3 sandwiches.

2. Cut the crusts off the sandwiches. Using a fork, press together the edges all the way around to seal.

3. Place the eggs in a shallow, wide bowl, and whisk in the milk.

4. Heat the oil and butter in a skillet over medium-high heat.

5. Gently dip the sandwiches into the egg mixture and flip, coating both sides and allowing the excess eggs to drip back into the bowl.

6. Carefully place the sandwiches into the skillet, cooking for about 2½ minutes per side (if all 3 sandwiches don't fit inside the skillet, cook them in batches). Remove from the skillet and cut in half.

7. While the sandwiches are cooking, warm the chutney or jam in a small saucepan on medium heat for 3 to 5 minutes or in the microwave on high for 30 seconds. Spoon over each and serve the Monte Cristo hot.

CALORIES **342**

TOTAL FAT **18 G**

CHOLESTEROL **147 MG**

SATURATED FAT **6 G**

TOTAL CARBOHYDRATES **26 G**

FIBER **3 G**

SUGAR **11 G**

SODIUM **152 MG**

PROTEIN **23 G**

Sloppy Joe

SERVES 6 (1 SANDWICH PER SERVING)

PREPARATION TIME **10 MINUTES**
COOKING TIME **25 TO 30 MINUTES**
TOTAL TIME **35 TO 40 MINUTES**

Using fresh, ripe tomatoes creates a brighter sauce, and adding carrots adds some natural sweetness without extra added sugar. This Joe is so sloppy that some people eat it with a fork and a knife.

1 tablespoon olive oil
2 carrots, peeled and chopped
½ cup cored, seeded, and chopped red or green bell pepper
½ cup chopped celery
1 medium red onion, chopped
8 whole sprigs fresh thyme
Fine-grained kosher salt and freshly ground black pepper, to taste
2 garlic cloves, minced
1½ pounds lean ground chicken or turkey
15 plum tomatoes or 10 vine-ripened or ripe beefsteak tomatoes
½ cup sugar-free ketchup
1 tablespoon Worcestershire sauce
2 tablespoons red wine vinegar
2 tablespoons brown sugar or brown sugar substitute of
    choice, divided
⅛ teaspoon ground cloves
2 teaspoons finely chopped fresh oregano
1 teaspoon ground cumin
⅛ teaspoon cayenne pepper (optional)
6 whole-wheat hamburger buns

1. Heat olive oil in a large sauté pan or skillet on medium heat.

2. Add the carrots, bell pepper, and celery, and sauté for 5 minutes. Reduce the heat if necessary. The vegetables should soften, but not brown.

3. Add the onion, thyme, and season with salt and pepper. Add 1 teaspoon of the brown sugar. Cook for 5 or so minutes, stirring occasionally and reducing the heat if necessary, until the onion caramelize a bit.

4. Add the garlic and cook for an additional 30 seconds, until golden and fragrant but not burnt. Remove from heat. Discard the thyme sprig stems (leaves should have fallen off). Transfer the vegetables to a bowl and set aside.

5. Reheat the pan on medium high. Put the ground poultry in the pan, and separate with the side of the wooden spoon to crumble. Cook for about 8 to 10 minutes, until browned, and no pink juices remain. Strain any fat. Add the vegetables back into the pan.

6. In a separate pot, combine the tomatoes, ketchup, Worcestershire sauce, vinegar, the rest of the brown sugar, cloves, oregano, cumin, and cayenne pepper, if using. Simmer over medium low heat for 10 minutes. Combine with the ground poultry and the vegetables and stir, heating for an additional 3 minutes until cooked through. Add more salt and pepper, if desired.

7. Open whole-wheat hamburger buns, and scoop a large amount of the Sloppy Joe mix into each bun. Close the buns and serve.

CALORIES **326**

TOTAL FAT **6 G**

CHOLESTEROL **81 MG**

SATURATED FAT **1 G**

TOTAL CARBOHYDRATES **45 G**

FIBER **5 G**

SUGAR **29 G**

SODIUM **208 MG**

PROTEIN **21 G**

Shrimp Po' Boy

SERVES 4

PREPARATION TIME **15 MINUTES**
COOKING TIME **5 TO 10 MINUTES**
TOTAL TIME **20 TO 25 MINUTES**

*A New Orleans classic, this sandwich is made with fried shrimp and a remou-
lade sauce, or spicy tartar sauce, and topped with shredded lettuce or cabbage.
The best kind of bread is a French baguette, but any kind of roll that has a
crunchy outside and a soft inside can work just as well.*

2 tablespoons brown mustard
1 cup nonfat mayonnaise
¼ cup nonfat Greek yogurt
1 tablespoon sweet pickle relish
1 teaspoon hot sauce
1 large garlic clove, minced
1 tablespoon ground paprika
1 teaspoon chili powder
1 teaspoon cayenne pepper
2 teaspoons fine-grained kosher salt, plus more, to taste
¾ cup fine cornmeal
¾ cup all-purpose flour
1 tablespoon Cajun seasoning
1 pound peeled and deveined medium shrimp
2 eggs, beaten, or ½ cup egg substitute
4 tablespoons canola oil
2 whole-wheat baguettes, halved, or 4 whole-wheat submarine buns
½ head iceberg lettuce or Napa cabbage, finely shredded
2 tomatoes, sliced

1. To make the remoulade, combine the mustard, mayonnaise, yogurt, relish,
hot sauce, garlic, paprika, chili powder, cayenne pepper, and a little salt. Set
aside in the refrigerator, so that the flavors can meld.

2. Meanwhile, combine the cornmeal, flour, Cajun seasoning, and 2 teaspoons
of salt in a shallow bowl. Set aside.

3. Dip the shrimp in the eggs, allowing any excess egg to drip back into the bowl, and then dredge the shrimp in the seasoned flour.

4. Warm up the oil in a sauté pan or skillet over medium-high heat, until it begins to shimmer but is not yet smoky. (If it starts to smoke, it's too hot, so remove it from heat.)

5. Pan-fry the dredged shrimp for about 2 minutes on each side, or until the shrimp has a crisp, golden coating. Remove the shrimp with tongs and place them on a plate covered with paper towels to absorb excess grease.

6. Open the bread lengthwise and spread the remoulade inside. Spread lettuce or Napa cabbage on the bottom of the roll, then top with the shrimp, and the sliced tomato. Serve while the shrimp is still warm.

CALORIES **239**

TOTAL FAT **15 G**

CHOLESTEROL **0 MG**

SATURATED FAT **1 G**

TOTAL CARBOHYDRATES **24 G**

FIBER **3 G**

SUGAR **4 G**

SODIUM **114 MG**

PROTEIN **4 G**

Philadelphia Cheesesteak

SERVES 8 (½ HOAGIE PER SERVING)

PREPARATION TIME **10 MINUTES**
COOKING TIME **15 MINUTES**
TOTAL TIME **25 MINUTES**

This recipe substitutes thinly cut deli roast beef for the usual raw beef, and is delicious when topped with melted cheese, bell pepper, onion, and mushrooms. If you're out of roast beef, deli-sliced turkey would be an acceptable alternative.

2 tablespoons olive oil
1 red or green bell pepper, cored, seeded, and cut into strips
1 large white onion, sliced
1 teaspoon Splenda or pinch of stevia powder or 2 to 4 drops stevia
    liquid concentrate
Fine-grained kosher salt and freshly ground black pepper, to taste
1 cup button mushrooms, sliced
16 slices deli-cut rare roast beef
2 garlic cloves, minced
6 slices provolone
4 tablespoons nonfat mayonnaise
4 whole-wheat hoagie rolls

1. Heat the olive oil in a sauté pan or skillet over medium heat. Add the bell pepper and cook for 3 to 5 minutes until softened, but not brown.

2. Add the onion and sweetener, season with salt and pepper, and cook for an additional 5 minutes until softened and translucent at the edges. Then add the mushrooms, and cook until all of the water has been released and evaporated, and the mushrooms are golden in color.

3. Add the roast beef and garlic and cook for 30 seconds. Remove from the heat, top the mixture with a single layer of the cheese slices, and cover the pan.

4. Spread mayonnaise on both sides of the rolls. Carefully place an even amount of beef and sautéed veggies into the rolls, leaving the melted cheese intact on top. Slice each hoagie in half on a diagonal.

CALORIES **258**

FIBER **1 G**

TOTAL FAT **8 G**

SUGAR **2 G**

CHOLESTEROL **38 MG**

SODIUM **229 MG**

SATURATED FAT **3 G**

PROTEIN **16 G**

TOTAL CARBOHYDRATES **10 G**

Turkey or Beef Burger with Special Sauce

SERVES 4

PREPARATION TIME **15 MINUTES**
COOKING TIME **10 MINUTES**
TOTAL TIME **25 MINUTES**

When craving one of those drive-through burgers that come in the cardboard box, take the time to make a fresh version instead, complete with tangy special sauce. You'll be in control of your sugar and salt intake, and will feel so much better afterwards.

1 pound lean ground turkey
1 teaspoon fine-grained kosher salt and 4 turns freshly ground black pepper, plus more, to taste
1 tablespoon olive oil
4 slices reduced-fat American cheese
2 tablespoons nonfat or low-fat salad dressing (such as low-fat Miracle Whip)
1½ tablespoons reduced-calorie French salad dressing
2 tablespoons nonfat mayonnaise
¼ tablespoon sweet pickle relish
¾ tablespoon dill pickle relish
½ teaspoon Splenda or 1 drop of stevia liquid concentrate
½ teaspoon dried onion flakes or ⅛ teaspoon onion powder
½ teaspoon white vinegar
½ teaspoon sugar-free ketchup
4 whole-wheat buns
1 cup shredded iceberg lettuce
8 dill pickle slices
½ cup finely chopped white onion

1. Combine the turkey with the salt and pepper, and form 8 turkey patties. Shape each patty with your hands by first making a ball and then flattening it and smoothing it around the edges.

2. Heat the olive oil in a large skillet or sauté pan, and add 3 or 4 patties and cook for 3 to 4 minutes. Flip the burgers and cook 2 minutes, then add the cheese and cover, cooking for an additional 2 minutes. Do not press on or poke the meat, and handle it carefully. The burgers are done when they are firm and the juices run clear.

3. Keep the cooked patties with cheese on a covered plate, and cook the second batch.

4. Meanwhile, prepare the special sauce by combining the salad dressings, mayonnaise, relishes, sweetener, onion flakes or powder, vinegar, and ketchup, and season with salt and pepper.

5. When you're ready to serve, place each burger on the bottom half of a bun and top with 1 tablespoon of the special sauce, shredded lettuce, 2 pickle slices, and finely chopped onion. Cover with the top of the bun.

CALORIES **354**

TOTAL FAT **15 G**

CHOLESTEROL **52 MG**

SATURATED FAT **3 G**

TOTAL CARBOHYDRATES **25 G**

FIBER **5 G**

SUGAR **11 G**

SODIUM **250 MG**

PROTEIN **28 G**

Cuban Sandwich

SERVES 4

PREPARATION TIME **5 MINUTES**
COOKING TIME **5 MINUTES**
TOTAL TIME **10 MINUTES**

Even though it's called a Cuban, this dish actually originates in Miami. Who knew that putting roast pork and ham in the same sandwich would make such a delicious combination?

4 whole-wheat hoagies or sandwich rolls
2 tablespoons yellow mustard
16 dill pickle slices
4 slices reduced-fat Swiss cheese
8 slices lean deli ham
4 slices roast pork
Canola oil cooking spray

1. Remove some of the bread from inside the hoagie or sandwich roll so that it's crustier and the sandwich is not too bready.

2. On one side of the hoagie or roll, spread a little mustard, place 4 pickle slices, 1 slice of Swiss cheese, 2 slices of ham folded in half and placed side by side, and a slice of roast pork. Spread a little more mustard on the other side of the hoagie or sandwich roll.

3. Cover a brick with foil or use a sandwich or Panini press (a waffle iron can also work). Spray the press, waffle iron, or sauté pan with cooking spray.

4. Flatten the sandwich with the press, waffle iron, or brick, and cook for 4 or 5 minutes, until the sandwich is crispy and the cheese is melted. If using the brick, flip the sandwich after 2 minutes. Serve hot.

CALORIES **314**
TOTAL FAT **7 G**
CHOLESTEROL **55 MG**
SATURATED FAT **5 G**
TOTAL CARBOHYDRATES **11 G**

FIBER **1 G**
SUGAR **1 G**
SODIUM **351 MG**
PROTEIN **19 G**

Open-Faced Tuna Melt

SERVES 4

PREPARATION TIME **10 MINUTES**
COOKING TIME **5 TO 10 MINUTES**
TOTAL TIME **15 TO 20 MINUTES**

Very creamy and satisfying, this classic diner-style grilled sandwich is high in protein. By making it open-faced, only one slice of bread is called for, reducing the total carbohydrates. Dig in!

1 tablespoon unsalted butter
4 slices rye or sourdough bread
2 (6-ounce) cans tuna in water, drained
¼ cup nonfat mayonnaise
Juice of ½ lemon
¼ cup chopped red onion
1 tablespoon capers, rinsed (optional)
2 tablespoons chopped fresh dill
Fine-grained kosher salt and freshly ground black pepper, to taste
4 slices tomato
4 slices reduced-fat sharp cheddar

1. Preheat the oven to 375 degrees F.

2. Butter one side of each bread slice, and place it on a nonstick or parchment-lined baking sheet.

3. In a medium bowl, combine the tuna, mayonnaise, lemon juice, onion, capers (if using), and dill. Season with salt and pepper, and mix until well incorporated.

4. Top each of the bread slices with a generous amount of the tuna salad, a tomato slice, and a slice of cheese.

5. Bake for 5 to 8 minutes until the cheese is melted and the bread is crisp and golden on the bottom. Serve immediately.

CALORIES **335**
TOTAL FAT **8 G**
CHOLESTEROL **63 MG**
SATURATED FAT **3 G**
TOTAL CARBOHYDRATES **22 G**

FIBER **5 G**
SUGAR **4 G**
SODIUM **318 MG**
PROTEIN **32 G**

Swiss and Mushroom Quesadilla

PREPARATION TIME **5 MINUTES**
COOKING TIME **5 TO 10 MINUTES**
TOTAL TIME **10 TO 15 MINUTES**

Melted cheese and mushrooms blend beautifully in this recipe. If you really want to go to town, serve these quesadillas with some sour cream, pico de gallo salsa, and guacamole. (To make an easy guacamole and pico de gallo salsa, see Breakfast Burrito on page 18.)

2 tablespoons olive oil, divided
1 pint (2 cups) button mushrooms, sliced
4 large whole-wheat flour tortillas or wraps
8 slices reduced-fat Swiss cheese
½ cup chopped cilantro or parsley for garnish (optional)
Fine-grained kosher salt and freshly ground black pepper, to taste

1. Heat 1 tablespoon of the olive oil in a sauté pan or skillet over medium heat, and add in the mushrooms. Cook until the mushrooms have released their water and it has evaporated, and the mushrooms are golden brown and tender.

2. Assemble the quesadillas by topping each of the tortillas with 2 cheese slices and mushrooms.

3. Add the remaining olive oil to the pan used for the mushrooms, and carefully place the first tortilla with the toppings in the pan. Cook flat until the cheese melts and the quesadilla is crisp. Fold the tortilla into a half circle, and remove. Repeat with the rest of the quesadillas.

4. Sprinkle the quesadillas with the cilantro or parsley (if using) and season with salt and pepper before serving.

CALORIES **282**
TOTAL FAT **5 G**
CHOLESTEROL **15 MG**
SATURATED FAT **1 G**
TOTAL CARBOHYDRATES **38 G**

FIBER **2 G**
SUGAR **2 G**
SODIUM **280 MG**
PROTEIN **22 G**

Soups and Stews (and Chili!)

CHAPTER SEVEN

Soups and Stews (and Chili!)

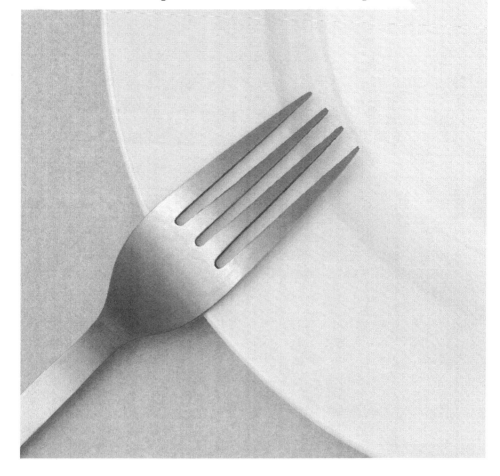

Cream of Tomato Soup

SERVES 6

PREPARATION TIME **5 MINUTES**
COOKING TIME **15 TO 20 MINUTES**
TOTAL TIME **20 TO 25 MINUTES**

Much better than the canned variety, this soup is fast and easy to make and tastes great with a grilled cheese sandwich. Basil and tomatoes make for a great combination, so if you've got some fresh basil, it'll really take your soup to a whole new level.

10 ripe tomatoes, chopped
6 to 8 cups homemade or commercial low-sodium vegetable or
    chicken stock
15 fresh basil leaves (optional)
1 cup nonfat half-and-half
Fine-grained kosher salt and freshly ground black pepper, to taste

1. In a soup pot, combine the tomatoes and stock and cook for 10 to 15 minutes over medium heat, until tomatoes are softened.

2. Purée the tomatoes with the stock, filling the blender halfway each time, and add fresh basil leaves, if using, to each batch. Return each batch to the pot, and then strain the purée through a fine mesh strainer to catch the tomato peels and seeds. Use the back of a ladle to press the soup through the strainer.

3. Return the strained soup to the pot. Cook over medium-low heat for 3 to 5 minutes, until hot. Reduce the heat to low, and stir in the nonfat half-and-half. Season with salt and pepper, and serve. Remove from the heat.

CALORIES **84**	FIBER **3 G**
TOTAL FAT **1 G**	SUGAR **7 G**
CHOLESTEROL **2 MG**	SODIUM **103 MG**
SATURATED FAT **0 G**	PROTEIN **5 G**
TOTAL CARBOHYDRATES **16 G**	

Hearty Beef Stew

SERVES 10

PREPARATION TIME **20 MINUTES**
COOKING TIME **2 HOURS 30 MINUTES**
TOTAL TIME **2 HOURS 50 MINUTES TO 3 HOURS 20 MINUTES**

Made with slow-stewed tender beef and hefty pieces of root vegetables and mushrooms, this hearty, rustic stew is ideal on a frigid winter day. This recipe works best when you have a good amount of time. Make it on a Sunday and have it for lunch during the week, or make it at night for dinner the next day.

1 pound beef chuck, chopped into 2-inch cubes
2 tablespoons vegetable oil
2 tablespoons all-purpose flour
Fine-grained kosher salt and freshly ground black pepper, to taste
2 tablespoons unsalted butter
2 medium white onions, chopped into large chunks
5 garlic cloves, minced
1 pint button mushrooms, halved
1 tablespoon tomato paste
9 cups homemade or commercial low-sodium beef stock
1 cup dry red wine
6 sprigs fresh thyme
4 sprigs fresh oregano
1 bay leaf
2 whole sprigs fresh rosemary
3 medium red potatoes, cut into large chunks
3 parsnips, peeled and cut into large chunks (optional)
4 medium carrots, peeled and cut into large chunks
2 celery stalks, chopped into large chunks
1 small can crushed tomatoes, fire-roasted preferred

1. Preheat the oven to 275 degrees F.

2. Pat the beef cubes dry with a paper towel so that there is no excess moisture on their surface.

3. Heat the oil in a Dutch oven or oven-safe soup pot with a tight-fitting lid over high heat until shimmering, but not smoking. (If the oil starts smoking during the cooking process, turn the heat down to medium.)

4. Meanwhile, spread the flour in an even layer on a plate. Season the beef cubes with salt and pepper and then coat all sides with the flour, shaking any excess flour off onto the plate.

5. Place the beef cubes in the oil so that they are in an even layer and not touching. (You may need to do this in two batches.) Brown well on all sides, for about 1 to 2 minutes a side, or for about 8 to 10 minutes altogether. Remove the pot from the heat, and take the beef cubes out with kitchen tongs or a slotted spoon, placing them on a plate. Discard any remaining oil.

6. Return the pot to the stove, and melt the butter over medium-high heat. Add the onion, and cook for about 5 minutes, or until translucent and softened.

7. Stir in the garlic, and cook for 30 seconds, until golden and fragrant.

8. Add the mushrooms, and cook until they turn golden in color.

9. Add the tomato paste, and cook for 1 minute more, until slightly browned.

10. Return the beef to the pot. Add the stock and red wine.

11. Tie the herb sprigs together with kitchen twine, and add them to the pot (if you don't have any twine, just put them in loosely, to be removed later).

12. Season with salt and a generous amount of black pepper.

13. Slow cook the meat in the oven for about 2 to 2½ hours, or until very tender.

14. After about 1 hour, or halfway through, stir in all of the remaining vegetables and crushed tomatoes and return the pot to the oven.

15. Remove the pot from the oven. Add 5 ice cubes to the top, wait for them to dissolve, and then skim the fat from the top with a spoon.

16. Remove the thyme and oregano sprigs and the bay leaf.

17. When ready to serve, simmer on low on the stove top. Season with more salt and pepper if needed.

18. Ladle into bowls. Serve with crusty whole-wheat, sourdough, or pumpernickel bread or rolls.

CALORIES **282**
TOTAL FAT **14 G**
CHOLESTEROL **47 MG**
SATURATED FAT **5 G**
TOTAL CARBOHYDRATES **25 G**

FIBER **7 G**
SUGAR **4 G**
SODIUM **182 MG**
PROTEIN **12 G**

Chicken Noodle Soup

SERVES 8

PREPARATION TIME **10 MINUTES**
COOKING TIME **20 MINUTES**
TOTAL TIME **30 MINUTES**

For comfort and simple nourishment, nothing can beat a traditional chicken noodle soup. However, if you're concerned about processed carbs, try making this soup with barley or instant brown rice (cooking time may need to be adjusted accordingly).

2 tablespoons olive oil
2 medium carrots, peeled and chopped
2 stalks celery, chopped
1 medium white onion, chopped
4 sprigs fresh thyme
1 bay leaf
3 garlic cloves, minced
2 quarts homemade or commercial low-sodium chicken stock
2 cups egg or soba noodles
2 cooked chicken breasts, skin removed and chopped
Fine-grained kosher salt and freshly ground black pepper, to taste
½ cup finely chopped parsley or cilantro, for garnish

1. Add the oil to the bottom of a large soup pot, and place over medium heat. Add the carrots and celery, and cook for about 5 minutes. Add the onion, thyme, and bay leaf, and cook for an additional 5 minutes. Lower the heat if necessary so as not to brown the vegetables. Add the minced garlic and cook for an additional 30 seconds.

2. Pour in the stock, stir, and turn the heat up to high to bring it to a boil. Just as the stock reaches a boil, reduce the heat to medium. Add the noodles. Let cook for 5 to 8 minutes.

3. Reduce the heat to low, add the chicken, and allow it to warm through, cooking for about 3 minutes.

4. Remove from the heat. Discard the thyme sprigs and bay leaf. Season with salt and pepper. Garnish with cilantro or parsley just prior to serving.

CALORIES **200**

TOTAL FAT **7 G**

CHOLESTEROL **47 MG**

SATURATED FAT **1 G**

TOTAL CARBOHYDRATES **14 G**

FIBER **2 G**

SUGAR **2 G**

SODIUM **124 MG**

PROTEIN **21 G**

Soups and Stews (and Chili!)

Herbed Minestrone

SERVES 8

PREPARATION TIME **10 MINUTES**
COOKING TIME **25 TO 30 MINUTES**
TOTAL TIME **35 TO 40 MINUTES**

This savory, tomato-based soup is brimming with Italian flavor. The elbow pasta and the kidney beans make this traditional soup very filling. The spinach is added at the very end, just prior to serving, so that it wilts slightly into the soup and retains its bright, fresh green color.

2 tablespoons olive oil
2 stalks celery, diced
1 large carrot, peeled and diced
1 large onion, diced
4 garlic cloves, minced
6 cups homemade or commercial low-sodium chicken stock
6 sprigs fresh oregano
6 sprigs fresh thyme
10 tomatoes or 15 plum tomatoes, peeled and coarsely chopped
⅓ pound green beans, trimmed and cut into ½-inch pieces (about 1½ cups)
1 cup whole-wheat elbow macaroni
1 (15-ounce) can kidney beans, drained and rinsed
½ cup chopped fresh basil
1 (10-ounce) package prewashed baby spinach
Fine-grained kosher salt and freshly ground black pepper, to taste
¼ cup finely grated Parmesan cheese, for garnish

1. Add the olive oil to the bottom of a soup pot over medium heat.

2. Add the celery and carrot, and cook for 5 to 8 minutes, or until they begin to soften.

3. Add the onion and cook for 4 to 6 minutes, or until the onion is softened and translucent at the edges. Add the garlic and cook for 30 seconds, until golden and fragrant but not burnt.

4. Add the chicken stock, fresh herb sprigs, tomatoes, green beans, and the macaroni to the pot and bring to a boil. Then reduce the heat to low and simmer for 10 minutes.

5. Add the kidney beans, chopped basil, and baby spinach, and cook for 3 minutes, or until beans are cooked through and spinach is wilted. Remove the herb sprigs and season with salt and pepper.

6. Serve in soup bowls and garnish with freshly grated Parmesan.

Peeling Tomatoes

If you don't want tomato skins floating in your minestrone, here's a quick way to peel them. Mark a large X with a paring knife in the bottom (blossom) end of each tomato, and drop them into boiling water for a few seconds; then remove with a slotted spoon and cool. The skin will easily peel off from where you made the cuts.

CALORIES **261**

TOTAL FAT **7 G**

CHOLESTEROL **3 MG**

SATURATED FAT **2 G**

TOTAL CARBOHYDRATES **42 G**

FIBER **13 G**

SUGAR **8 G**

SODIUM **296 MG**

PROTEIN **13 G**

Turkey Chili with Cinnamon and Cocoa

SERVES 8

PREPARATION TIME **10 MINUTES**
COOKING TIME **40 MINUTES TO 1 HOUR**
TOTAL TIME **50 MINUTES TO 1 HOUR 10 MINUTES**

Turkey chili is warmed up and sweetened slightly with added cinnamon and cocoa. Both ingredients pair extremely well with the chiles in this dish. Rather than just chili powder, actual chiles are used. Have a heaping bowl. It's good for you, too!

Dress this chili up with a topping of chopped scallions, cilantro, or parsley and a dollop of nonfat Greek yogurt (or nonfat sour cream). Grated, low-fat cheddar cheese can be sprinkled on, if desired.

2 to 3 chiles de arbol, stem and seeds removed
5 ancho chiles, stem and seeds removed
10 plum tomatoes, fire roasted or raw, coarsely chopped
2 tablespoons olive oil
1 medium to large yellow or white onion, chopped
1 pound ground turkey
3 cups freshly cooked or low-sodium canned black beans,
    rinsed and drained
2½ cups chicken or vegetable stock
2 teaspoons dried oregano
2 teaspoons ground cumin
1 tablespoon unsweetened cocoa powder
½ teaspoon ground cinnamon
Fine-grained kosher salt, to taste

1. Toast chiles in sauté pan over medium heat for 2 minutes on both sides, or until fragrant.

2. Purée the plum tomatoes and toasted chiles in a blender, and strain through a fine mesh strainer to catch skins and seeds.

3. Heat the olive oil and onion in a soup pan until the onion is cooked through and translucent at the edges.

4. Add the ground turkey, and cook for 10 to 15 minutes over medium heat until turkey is cooked through.

5. Add the beans, puréed tomato and chile mixture, stock, oregano, cumin, cocoa powder, and cinnamon to the meat.

6. Cook for 20 to 30 minutes over medium-low heat until flavors are combined and chili is hot. Season with salt, and serve immediately.

CALORIES **329**

TOTAL FAT **10 G**

CHOLESTEROL **77 MG**

SATURATED FAT **2 G**

TOTAL CARBOHYDRATES **33 G**

FIBER **11 G**

SUGAR **6 G**

SODIUM **220 MG**

PROTEIN **29 G**

Soups and Stews (and Chili!)

Potato Corn Chowder

PREPARATION TIME **15 MINUTES**
COOKING TIME **40 MINUTES**
TOTAL TIME **55 MINUTES**

This creamy vegetarian chowder makes use of corncobs in the stock, lending a sweeter, richer corn flavor to the soup. Basil adds some brightness to the soup, and cornstarch is used to thicken the stock.

4 potatoes, peeled and cubed
3 corncobs, kernels cut off, cobs reserved
½ leek, sliced
2 cups homemade or commercial low-sodium chicken or
    vegetable stock
2 cups cold water
2 tablespoons cornstarch or tapioca starch
½ cup 1 percent milk
Fine-grained kosher salt and freshly ground black pepper, to taste
¼ cup chopped fresh basil

1. Put the potatoes, corn kernels, corncobs, leek, chicken or vegetable stock, and cold water in a large soup pot on the stove top, and bring to a boil over high heat. Reduce to medium heat, and cook for 5 additional minutes or until potatoes are cooked through and can be pierced with a fork easily.

2. Remove the corncobs.

3. Remove about 1 cup of the potatoes and purée them in the blender on medium until a paste is formed. Alternately, use a hand blender in the soup to purée some of the potatoes.

4. Make a slurry by whisking the starch into the milk until fully combined. Add the milk slurry and potato purée (if a standing blender was used) to the soup. Stir constantly over medium-high heat for 5 more minutes or until thickened. If the soup is not as thick as desired, simply purée some more of the potatoes and stir well to combine.

5. Remove from the heat. Season with salt and pepper, and stir in the chopped basil before serving.

CALORIES **184**

TOTAL FAT **2 G**

CHOLESTEROL **2 MG**

SATURATED FAT **1 G**

TOTAL CARBOHYDRATES **38 G**

FIBER **5 G**

SUGAR **5 G**

SODIUM **261 MG**

PROTEIN **7 G**

Soups and Stews (and Chili!)

Creamy Mushroom Soup

SERVES 6 TO 8

PREPARATION TIME **20 MINUTES**
COOKING TIME **30 MINUTES**
TOTAL TIME **50 MINUTES**

This familiar recipe can be made with a twist—by using almond milk, which tastes really great with mushrooms. With the fresh herbs adding extra flavor, this soup will be worth the time you take to prepare it.

2 shallots or ½ white onion, finely chopped
4 tablespoons olive oil, divided
2 garlic cloves, minced
2 cups button mushrooms, sliced
1 teaspoon finely chopped fresh oregano
8 fresh thyme sprigs
1 teaspoon minced fresh rosemary sprigs, woody stems discarded
2 tablespoons dry white wine or 1 tablespoon vinegar
6 tablespoons all-purpose flour
2½ cups unsweetened almond milk or 1 percent milk
2 cups homemade or commercial low-sodium mushroom, vegetable, beef, or chicken stock
Fine-grained kosher salt and freshly ground black pepper, to taste
¼ cup chopped fresh parsley for garnish (optional)

1. In the bottom of a soup pot, saute the shallots or onion with 2 tablespoons of the olive oil over medium heat, stirring occasionally, until softened and translucent, or for about 5 minutes.

2. Add the garlic and cook for 30 more seconds.

3. Add the mushrooms, oregano, thyme, and rosemary, and cook for an additional 6 to 8 minutes, until mushrooms have lost their liquid and it has evaporated, and they are golden in color. Remove the thyme stems.

4. Add the wine or the vinegar, return to medium-high heat, and scrape the bits from the bottom of the pan with a wooden spoon. Allow some of the liquid to evaporate, cooking for 3 minutes. Empty the mixture into a bowl.

5. In the bottom of the soup pot, add the rest of the olive oil and whisk in the flour immediately. Whisk constantly for 4 to 5 minutes over medium-low heat to form a golden paste with a nutty fragrance.

6. Gradually add the milk to the paste, whisking constantly for about 5 minutes until a thick cream is formed.

7. Add the stock to the sauce, and cook for 3 minutes more until hot. Add the cooked vegetables back into the pot and stir.

8. Season with salt and pepper, and garnish with parsley, if desired.

CALORIES **188**

TOTAL FAT **10 G**

CHOLESTEROL **6 MG**

SATURATED FAT **2 G**

TOTAL CARBOHYDRATES **20 G**

FIBER **2 G**

SUGAR **6 G**

SODIUM **181 MG**

PROTEIN **6 G**

Soups and Stews (and Chili!)

Autumn Squash and Carrot Soup

SERVES 8 TO 10

PREPARATION TIME **20 MINUTES**
COOKING TIME **30 TO 35 MINUTES**
TOTAL TIME **50 TO 55 MINUTES**

This sweet and luscious soup is perfect for a fall lunch or dinner. Adding apples creates a deeper flavor. To peel butternut squash, first split the vegetable in half with a chef's knife, scoop out the seeds, and then split it in half again. Use a vegetable peeler to remove the skin, holding the squash steady on its flat side.

2 tablespoons olive oil
1 medium to large white onion, coarsely chopped
2 garlic cloves, minced
1 butternut squash or 2 acorn squash, peeled, seeded, and
    coarsely chopped
2 Granny Smith or similar apples, peeled, cored, and chopped
1 medium starchy potato such as Idaho (also called Russet)
4 carrots, peeled and coarsely chopped
6 to 8 cups homemade or commercial low-sodium vegetable or
    chicken stock
1 bay leaf
1 teaspoon mild yellow curry powder (optional)
2-inch piece fresh gingerroot, juiced (see page 74), or 1 teaspoon
    ground ginger
2 tablespoons fresh lemon juice
Fine-grained kosher salt, to taste

1. In the bottom of a soup pot or Dutch oven, heat the olive oil and add onion. Cook for 5 minutes, or until the onion are softened and translucent.

2. Add the garlic and cook for 30 seconds longer, until it is golden and fragrant but not burned.

3. Add the squash, apples, potatoes, carrots, and enough stock to cover them by a few inches. Add the bay leaf and the curry powder, if using, and bring the mixture to a boil over high heat.

4. Turn down to medium heat to simmer and loosely cover, cooking for about 20 to 25 minutes, until all of the vegetables are cooked through and softened.

5. In a standing blender in batches, filling halfway each time, and holding the lid with a kitchen towel, purée the soup. Add purée back to the pot after each batch. Alternately, use an immersion blender (also called a hand or stick blender) directly in the pot, puréeing all of the soup.

6. Once the soup is puréed, add more stock if necessary to achieve desired consistency. Add the ginger and lemon juice, and stir. Season with salt, and serve immediately.

CALORIES **200**

TOTAL FAT **3 G**

CHOLESTEROL **2 MG**

SATURATED FAT **1 G**

TOTAL CARBOHYDRATES **39 G**

FIBER **6 G**

SUGAR **9 G**

SODIUM **160 MG**

PROTEIN **6 G**

Soups and Stews (and Chili!)

Thai Red Curry Noodle Soup

SERVES 6

PREPARATION TIME **15 MINUTES**
COOKING TIME **20 MINUTES**
TOTAL TIME **35 MINUTES**

This spicy noodle soup is great in hot or cold weather. If you can find it, curry paste is preferable to curry powder. Soba noodles are buckwheat noodles and can be found in the Asian section of grocery stores or in health food stores. You may not have fish sauce handy, either, but it will add authentic flavor to your soup. Just don't be put off by the pungent smell when you crack it open!

2 teaspoons olive oil
2 tablespoons Thai red curry paste or 3 tablespoons red
    curry powder
8 cups homemade or commercial low-sodium vegetable or
    chicken stock
2 tablespoons fish sauce (optional)
2 tablespoons brown sugar or brown sugar substitute
Juice of 2 limes
1-inch piece fresh gingerroot, halved
8 ounces Thai-style rice noodles, brown rice noodles, soba noodles,
    or thin whole-wheat spaghetti
1 cooked chicken breast (skin removed), shredded
Fine-grained kosher salt, to taste
¼ cup chopped fresh basil leaves for garnish
¼ cup chopped fresh cilantro for garnish
¼ cup sliced scallions for garnish

1. Heat the olive oil in the bottom of a large soup pot, and add in the curry, whisking to incorporate with the oil. Whisk in the stock, fish sauce, sweetener, and lime juice, and bring to a boil. Add the pieces of gingerroot. Then reduce the heat to medium low and simmer for 10 to 15 minutes.

2. Meanwhile, cook the noodles separately according to the package directions. Drain and rinse in hot water.

3. Stir the noodles and the shredded chicken into the soup. Remove from the heat. Season with salt.

4. Ladle into bowls, and garnish with the cilantro, basil, and scallions before serving.

CALORIES **214**

TOTAL FAT **2 G**

CHOLESTEROL **3 MG**

SATURATED FAT **0 G**

TOTAL CARBOHYDRATES **26 G**

FIBER **2 G**

SUGAR **6 G**

SODIUM **133 MG**

PROTEIN **5 G**

Soups and Stews (and Chili!)

Fresh Pea Soup

SERVES 6

PREPARATION TIME **10 MINUTES**
COOKING TIME **15 TO 20 MINUTES**
TOTAL TIME **25 TO 30 MINUTES**

This puréed soup is very bright green as long as you use good-quality peas. It's a little counterintuitive, but flash-frozen peas are often preferable to fresh peas found in the vegetable section. The peas are frozen when exactly ripe and tender, whereas sometimes fresh peas can be chalky because they are only at their peak for a limited amount of time and turn quickly.

This soup tastes great whether served cool or warmed. It's a little taste of summer, whether or not it's hot outside.

1 tablespoon olive oil
1 medium white onion, coarsely chopped
2 to 3 cups homemade or commercial low-sodium chicken or
    vegetable stock
5 small fresh mint sprigs
1 (10-ounce) bag good-quality frozen peas
Fine-grained kosher salt, to taste
1 tablespoon fresh lemon juice
4 tablespoons nonfat Greek yogurt or nonfat sour cream for garnish
¼ cup chopped chives or parsley for garnish (optional)

1. Heat olive oil in a large soup pot over medium heat, add the onion and cook until translucent and tender. Add the stock, mint, and peas, and heat until just cooked through.

2. In a standing blender in batches, filling halfway each time, and holding the top of the blender with a kitchen towel, purée until smooth. Alternately, use an immersion blender (also called a stick or hand blender) to purée the soup in the pot. Season with salt, and stir.

3. Serve the soup hot, or chill and serve cold. To chill the soup, place it in a bowl inside a larger bowl filled with ice and some cold water. Stir occasionally to speed cooling. Once cool, refrigerate to chill further.

4. Just prior to serving, stir in the lemon juice. Ladle into bowls, and garnish each soup with a dollop of yogurt or sour cream. Sprinkle on chives or parsley, if desired.

CALORIES **133**

TOTAL FAT **4 G**

CHOLESTEROL **45 MG**

SATURATED FAT **1 G**

TOTAL CARBOHYDRATES **6 G**

FIBER **1 G**

SUGAR **3 G**

SODIUM **91 MG**

PROTEIN **17 G**

Soups and Stews (and Chili!)

Herbed Lentil Soup

SERVES 10

PREPARATION TIME **15 MINUTES**
COOKING TIME **45 MINUTES**
TOTAL TIME **1 HOUR**

Lentils are a dried legume that comes in a variety of sizes and colors and are high in protein, dietary fiber, and a number of essential vitamins and minerals. This deliciously herbed lentil soup is served puréed, but if you prefer a chunkier version, skip the blending and enjoy the texture of the whole lentils.

2 tablespoons olive oil
2 medium carrots, peeled and finely chopped
2 ribs celery, finely chopped
Fine-grained kosher salt, to taste
1 medium white onion, finely chopped
2 garlic cloves, minced
2¼ cups dry green or red lentils, picked through and rinsed
1 (8-ounce) can crushed tomatoes
2 quarts homemade or commercial low-sodium chicken or
    vegetable stock
½ tablespoon minced fresh rosemary
½ tablespoon minced fresh oregano
1 tablespoon fresh thyme
6 tablespoons nonfat sour cream or nonfat Greek yogurt
½ cup finely chopped chives for garnish (optional)

1. Heat the olive oil in a soup pot over medium heat. Add the carrots and celery, and season with salt, and cook for 5 minutes. Add the onion and cook for an additional 5 minutes until it is softened and translucent. Add the garlic and cook for an additional 30 seconds until it is golden and fragrant but not burnt.

2. Stir in the lentils, tomatoes, stock, and herbs. Increase to high heat to bring to a boil, and then reduce the heat to low and allow to simmer covered until the lentils are softened, or for about 35 minutes.

3. Purée the soup in batches in a standing blender, filling only halfway each time and holding the lid with a kitchen towel. Alternately, use an immersion blender (also called a hand or stick blender) to purée the soup in the pot.

4. Ladle the soup into individual bowls, and top with a dollop of sour cream or yogurt. Garnish with chives, if using.

CALORIES **329**

TOTAL FAT **4 G**

CHOLESTEROL **89 MG**

SATURATED FAT **1 G**

TOTAL CARBOHYDRATES **31 G**

FIBER **15 G**

SUGAR **3 G**

SODIUM **200 MG**

PROTEIN **55 G**

Soups and Stews (and Chili!)

Vegetable Side Dishes

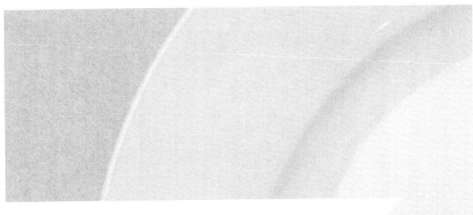

Vegetable Side Dishes

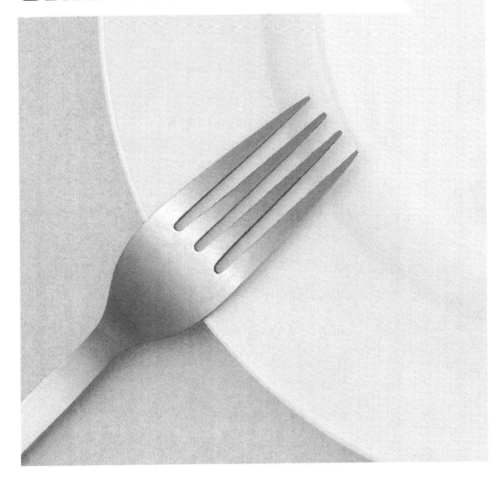

Creamed Spinach

SERVES 6

PREPARATION TIME **5 MINUTES**
COOKING TIME **10 MINUTES**
TOTAL TIME **15 MINUTES**

This recipe offers the perfect way to get one's greens into a meal. Use prewashed and packaged baby spinach to cut down on preparation time, and you'll have smooth and creamy spinach to serve as a great side dish with chicken or pork.

2 tablespoons olive oil, divided
1 medium red onion or 2 shallots, finely chopped
Fine-grained kosher salt, to taste
1 tablespoon all-purpose flour
½ cup 1 percent milk
⅛ teaspoon freshly grated nutmeg
½ teaspoon ground white pepper or pinch of cayenne pepper
2 (10-ounce) packages prewashed baby spinach
2 tablespoons freshly grated Parmesan cheese

1. Heat 1 tablespoon of the olive oil in a sauté pan over medium heat, and add in the onion or shallots and season with salt. Cook for 5 minutes or until the onion is softened and translucent at the edges.

2. Add the rest of the olive oil and the flour, and whisk constantly for 3 minutes until a golden, nutty-smelling paste is formed. (Just whisk the onion or shallots with the paste; there's no need to remove them from pan.)

3. Slowly pour in the milk while whisking constantly. Add the nutmeg and the white or cayenne pepper, and continue to whisk until a thick sauce is formed.

4. Add the baby spinach to the hot sauce, and stir until wilted. Serve hot, sprinkled with Parmesan cheese.

CALORIES **91**
TOTAL FAT **7 G**
CHOLESTEROL **3 MG**
SATURATED FAT **2 G**
TOTAL CARBOHYDRATES **4 G**

FIBER **0 G**
SUGAR **2 G**
SODIUM **282 MG**
PROTEIN **2 G**

Creamed Corn

SERVES 6

PREPARATION TIME **5 MINUTES**
COOKING TIME **10 TO 20 MINUTES**
TOTAL TIME **15 TO 25 MINUTES**

*Sweet corn kernels become very velvety when puréed with this creamy sauce.
If using frozen corn, remember to thaw it out ahead of time for this recipe. If
it's summertime and fresh corn is available, use that instead—just remove the
husks, break each cob in half, and, placing it vertically on the cutting board,
cut off the kernels from each side using a sharp knife.*

1 tablespoon olive oil
1 tablespoon all-purpose flour
½ cup 1 percent milk
2 (16-ounce) packages frozen corn kernels, thawed, or 4 cups fresh
    corn kernels cut from the cob
½ cup fresh, finely chopped basil (optional)
1 tablespoon mascarpone cheese or 1 tablespoon unsalted butter
Fine-grained kosher salt, to taste
¼ teaspoon paprika for garnish (optional)

1. Add the olive oil and the flour to the bottom of a medium saucepan over
medium heat and whisk constantly for 3 minutes until a golden, nutty-
smelling paste is formed.

2. Pour in the milk and whisk constantly. Add the corn kernels and cook on
low for about 5 minutes, until cooked through.

3. Using an immersion blender (also called a stick or hand blender), purée
the corn in the pot. Alternately, transfer the corn mixture to a stand blender
in batches, filling only halfway each time and puréeing for only 30 seconds
or less. The corn should be just slightly puréed, not totally smooth.

4. Stir in the chopped fresh basil, if using. Remove from the heat, and add
in the mascarpone or butter. Season with salt. Sprinkle with a dusting of
paprika to add color and flavor, if using. Serve hot.

CALORIES **94**
TOTAL FAT **3 G**
CHOLESTEROL **3 MG**
SATURATED FAT **1 G**
TOTAL CARBOHYDRATES **16 G**

FIBER **2 G**
SUGAR **3 G**
SODIUM **261 MG**
PROTEIN **3 G**

Sour Cream Mashed Potatoes

SERVES 8

PREPARATION TIME **10 MINUTES**
COOKING TIME **25 TO 30 MINUTES (INCLUDING BOILING WATER)**
TOTAL TIME **35 TO 40 MINUTES**

This is a classic recipe for a dish that is a perfect side for just about any entrée, from Thanksgiving turkey to rotisserie chicken, pork chops, and vegetarian entrées as well. The sour cream is the secret ingredient here that will make the potatoes creamy, tangy, and satisfying. But don't overmix them, or they will turn gluey.

3 pounds waxy potatoes such as Yukon gold or round white, peeled
    and chopped into large pieces
2 teaspoons fine-grained kosher salt, divided, plus more to taste
2 tablespoons unsalted butter
1½ cups 1 percent milk or lowfat buttermilk
1 cup nonfat sour cream
Freshly ground black pepper, to taste

1. Add the potatoes to a pot and cover with cold water. Add 2 teaspoons of salt. Place the pot over high heat and bring to a boil.

2. Cook the potatoes for 15 to 20 minutes, until tender (test by piercing with a fork or sharp knife), and drain them in a colander.

3. To mash the potatoes, use a food mill, a potato ricer, a potato masher, or the paddle attachment on the stand mixer.

4. While mashing, add the butter, milk or buttermilk, and the sour cream and combine, but don't overmix. Season with salt and pepper, and serve.

CALORIES **182**
TOTAL FAT **3 G**
CHOLESTEROL **12 MG**
SATURATED FAT **2 G**
TOTAL CARBOHYDRATES **34 G**

FIBER **4 G**
SUGAR **4 G**
SODIUM **112 MG**
PROTEIN **5 G**

Sweet Potato Casserole

SERVES 10

PREPARATION TIME **20 MINUTES**
COOKING TIME **20 MINUTES TO 1 HOUR (DEPENDING WHETHER MICROWAVE OR OVEN IS USED TO COOK SWEET POTATOES)**
TOTAL TIME **40 MINUTES TO 1 HOUR 20 MINUTES**

This casserole is a popular Thanksgiving side dish, but it can be made for other occasions or as a family dinner side dish, not only for "turkey day." Imitation maple syrup used for creating this recipe can be found in many grocery stores.

6 medium to large sweet potatoes
1 cup whole pecans
2 tablespoons brown sugar or brown sugar substitute
2 teaspoons cinnamon
Pinch of fine-grained kosher salt, plus more, to taste
1 tablespoon unsalted butter
1 tablespoon sugar-free imitation maple syrup or sugar-free imitation honey
1 teaspoon pure vanilla extract
½ teaspoon freshly grated nutmeg or ½ teaspoon ground nutmeg
1 egg
Olive oil cooking spray

1. Preheat the oven to 400 degrees F.

2. Pierce each of the sweet potatoes several times with a fork, and bake for about 45 minutes or until tender. Alternately, cook the pierced yams on the high setting in the microwave for 10 minutes. Stop halfway through to check the yams and adjust time accordingly, if necessary. Rotate the yams if necessary. Set aside to cool for about 10 minutes.

3. Grind the pecans in a food processor or blender. Add the sweetener, cinnamon, pinch of salt, and butter, and process until blended.

4. Cut the sweet potatoes in half, and scoop out the flesh, discarding the skins. Purée the sweet potatoes in a blender or food processor. Add the maple syrup or honey, vanilla, and nutmeg. Add in the egg and purée. Season with salt.

5. Spray a baking dish with olive oil cooking spray. Add the sweet potato purée, and sprinkle the pecan topping on. Bake for 10 to 15 minutes, or until the topping is crisp and has browned. Serve hot.

CALORIES **169**

TOTAL FAT **9 G**

CHOLESTEROL **19 MG**

SATURATED FAT **2 G**

TOTAL CARBOHYDRATES **21 G**

FIBER **4 G**

SUGAR **7 G**

SODIUM **50 MG**

PROTEIN **3 G**

Broccoli Casserole

SERVES 6

PREPARATION TIME **10 MINUTES**
COOKING TIME **30 TO 35 MINUTES**
TOTAL TIME **40 TO 45 MINUTES**

Buttery. Cheesy. Creamy. Yes, this broccoli casserole is the ideal comfort food, but it's also surprisingly good for you. Broccoli is a great source of protein and vitamin C, among a number of other vitamins and minerals, and very low in carbs. So dig in!

1 bunch broccoli florets, stalk discarded
6 ounces nonfat cream cheese, softened
½ cup reduced-fat sharp cheddar cheese
Fine-grained kosher salt and freshly ground black pepper, to taste
¼ cup whole-wheat bread crumbs
½ teaspoon dried oregano
½ teaspoon dried basil
1 tablespoon unsalted butter, melted
Olive oil cooking spray

1. Preheat the oven to 300 degrees F.

2. Bring a pot of salted water to a boil, and add the broccoli florets. Boil for 5 minutes or so to blanch. Broccoli should be bright green and tender but with some bite to it.

3. Remove the broccoli from the water with a slotted spoon or drain it in a colander.

4. In a large bowl, mix the cream cheese and cheddar cheese with the broccoli. Season with salt and pepper.

5. In a small bowl, mix together the bread crumbs with the dried herbs, season with salt and pepper, and add the butter to form a crumble.

6. Spray a baking dish with the cooking spray just to coat. Add the broccoli and sprinkle with the topping to cover.

7. Bake for about 25 to 30 minutes, or until top is browned and bubbling.

CALORIES **149**

TOTAL FAT **7 G**

CHOLESTEROL **20 MG**

SATURATED FAT **4 G**

TOTAL CARBOHYDRATES **13 G**

FIBER **3 G**

SUGAR **4 G**

SODIUM **141 MG**

PROTEIN **11 G**

Green Bean Casserole

SERVES 8

PREPARATION TIME **10 MINUTES**
COOKING TIME **30 MINUTES**
TOTAL TIME **40 MINUTES**

Savory mushrooms and sour cream come together to coat crispy green beans topped with crunchy baked onion slices. This version is the real thing—much richer in flavor than the canned concoction.

2 medium white onions, sliced very thinly, divided
¼ cup all-purpose flour
½ teaspoon fine-grained kosher salt
1 pound green beans, ends trimmed
6 sprigs fresh thyme
1 tablespoon olive oil
1 pint button mushrooms, sliced
2 garlic cloves, minced
½ cup homemade or commercial low-sodium chicken stock
½ cup nonfat sour cream

1. Preheat the oven to 350 degrees F.

2. Combine half of the onion slices with the flour and salt in a small bowl, and toss to coat. Place on a nonstick or parchment-lined baking sheet (nonstick preferred). Set aside.

3. Over high heat, bring a pot of salted water to a boil. Boil the green beans until bright green and tender, yet still crispy. Remove the beans with a slotted spoon, or drain in a colander. Submerge the beans in a large bowl of icy water so they retain their color and crispness. Set aside.

4. Heat the remaining onion slices and the thyme sprigs in olive oil over medium heat. Add the mushrooms and cook until the liquid is released and evaporated and they are golden. Add the garlic and cook for an additional 30 seconds. Add the chicken stock, and cook for about 3 minutes more over high heat, until most of the liquid has evaporated.

The Diabetic Cookbook

5. Combine the green beans with the mushroom mixture, and stir in the sour cream until well combined.

6. Pour the green bean mixture into a baking dish or pie pan. Bake the casserole and the crisp onion slices, separately, for about 15 minutes, until the casserole is bubbly and the onions are golden and crisp. Top the casserole with the crispy onion slices and serve.

CALORIES **102**

TOTAL FAT **5 G**

CHOLESTEROL **60 MG**

SATURATED FAT **2 G**

TOTAL CARBOHYDRATES **13 G**

FIBER **4 G**

SUGAR **2 G**

SODIUM **170 MG**

PROTEIN **3 G**

Vegetable Side Dishes

Collard Greens

SERVES 8

PREPARATION TIME **10 MINUTES**
COOKING TIME **2 HOURS**
TOTAL TIME **2 HOURS 10 MINUTES**

Greens are traditionally slow cooked to be meltingly tender. To give them a smoky, robust flavor, collard greens are generally cooked with a piece of meat. This recipe calls for turkey wings, but you may also use smoked ham hocks or even a little bacon.

1 medium white onion, finely chopped
2 tablespoons olive oil
3 garlic cloves, minced
8 cups homemade or commercial low-sodium chicken or
    turkey stock
2 smoked turkey wings
2 cups water
1 large bunch collard greens
1 tablespoon hot sauce
¼ cup apple cider vinegar
1 tablespoon unsalted butter
Fine-grained kosher salt and freshly ground black pepper, to taste

1. In the bottom of a large pot, cook the onion in olive oil over medium heat until it is translucent and softened, about 6 minutes. Add the garlic and cook for 30 seconds longer until golden and fragrant but not burnt.

2. Add the stock, turkey wings, and water, and bring just to a boil. Reduce heat to medium, and simmer ingredients covered for 1 hour.

3. Meanwhile, remove the tough stems from the collard greens by holding the greens in one hand and running the other hand down the stem. Another way is to cut the stem out with a knife.

4. Fill a clean sink or a large bowl with water and soak the collard greens, swishing the water to remove the grit.

5. Drain the greens and put them in the pot with the stock. Add the hot sauce, apple cider vinegar, and butter. Simmer uncovered, stirring occasionally, for about 50 minutes, or until greens are meltingly tender. Season with salt and pepper.

6. Strain the greens, reserving the liquid, which can be used for dipping or as a soup base.

CALORIES **244**

TOTAL FAT **6 G**

CHOLESTEROL **121 MG**

SATURATED FAT **2 G**

TOTAL CARBOHYDRATES **2 G**

FIBER **1 G**

SUGAR **3 G**

SODIUM **350 MG**

PROTEIN **44 G**

Spaghetti Squash

SERVES 6

PREPARATION TIME **3 MINUTES**
COOKING TIME **6 TO 40 MINUTES (DEPENDING ON WHETHER USING MICROWAVE OR OVEN)**
TOTAL TIME **9 TO 43 MINUTES**

Spaghetti squash is a great extremely low-calorie, zero-carbohydrate alternative to a pasta side. Grated Parmesan can be sprinkled on the strands before serving, if desired.

1 spaghetti squash
1 tablespoon olive oil
Fine-grained kosher salt and freshly ground black pepper, to taste

1. If baking the squash, preheat the oven to 375 degrees F.

2. Halve the spaghetti squash. Scoop out the seeds and pulp from the center of each half.

3. Coat each half with olive oil, and season with salt and pepper.

4. Place the squash halves on an ungreased baking sheet, peel-side down.

5. Bake for 35 to 40 minutes, or until tender when pierced with a fork or knife tip. (Alternately, microwave each oiled and seasoned squash half on a plate for 6 to 8 minutes on high.)

6. When the squash is cooked, separate the strands by running a fork through the vegetable to achieve a spaghetti-like dish.

CALORIES **22**
TOTAL FAT **2 G**
CHOLESTEROL **0 MG**
SATURATED FAT **0 G**
TOTAL CARBOHYDRATES **0 G**

FIBER **0 G**
SUGAR **0 G**
SODIUM **1 MG**
PROTEIN **0 G**

Succotash

PREPARATION TIME **3 MINUTES**
COOKING TIME **15 MINUTES**
TOTAL TIME **18 MINUTES**

This recipe will help you create the classic Southern side dish, using lima beans, corn, and butter. Fast and easy, it's full of flavor and is very filling.

3 cups frozen lima beans
4 cups fresh corn kernels cut from the cob or frozen corn kernels
2 tablespoons unsalted butter
Fine-grained kosher salt and freshly ground black pepper, to taste

1. Cook the lima beans in boiling salted water for about 10 minutes, or until almost tender.

2. Add the corn and cook for 5 minutes longer. Drain. Add the butter and stir well. Season with salt and pepper, and serve.

CALORIES **165**
TOTAL FAT **4 G**
CHOLESTEROL **8 MG**
SATURATED FAT **2 G**
TOTAL CARBOHYDRATES **28 G**

FIBER **5 G**
SUGAR **6 G**
SODIUM **77 MG**
PROTEIN **7 G**

Vegetable Side Dishes

Glazed Carrots

PREPARATION TIME **5 MINUTES**
COOKING TIME **25 MINUTES**
TOTAL TIME **30 MINUTES**

These glazed carrots are such a yummy vegetable side dish. You won't believe you can enjoy them guilt-free when the sweet tooth starts calling.

1 pound baby carrots
2 tablespoons unsalted butter
2 tablespoons imitation honey or brown sugar substitute
1 tablespoon fresh lemon juice
Fine-grained kosher salt, to taste

1. Bring water to a boil in a medium saucepan. Add the carrots and cook just until tender.

2. Drain the carrots and add them back to the pan with the butter, honey or brown sugar substitute, and lemon juice. Cook until a glaze coats the carrots, about 5 minutes. Season with more salt, if desired.

CALORIES **82**

TOTAL FAT **4 G**

CHOLESTEROL **10 MG**

SATURATED FAT **2 G**

TOTAL CARBOHYDRATES **12 G**

FIBER **2 G**

SUGAR **9 G**

SODIUM **217 MG**

PROTEIN **1 G**

Vegetarian Entrées

Vegetarian Entrées

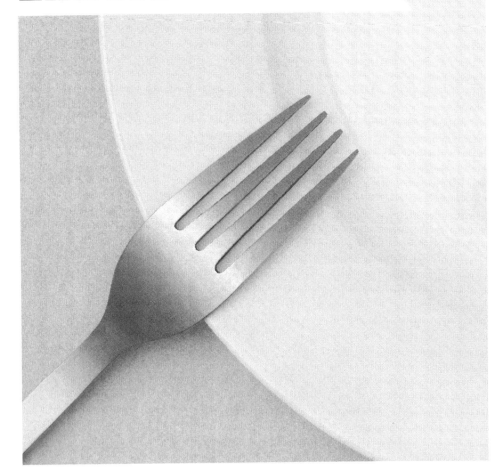

Quinoa and Vegetable-Stuffed Avocados

SERVES 4

PREPARATION TIME **10 MINUTES**
COOKING TIME **16 MINUTES**
TOTAL TIME **26 MINUTES**

New to quinoa? It's actually a seed with a springy, light, and grainlike texture. You'll find it in most grocery stores. In this dish, the quinoa is first toasted to bring out its nutty flavor. And it's simply delicious in this recipe!

½ cup uncooked quinoa
1½ teaspoons olive oil
1 cup cold water
½ cup chopped tomato
½ cup cored, seeded, and chopped red or yellow bell pepper
½ cup frozen or fresh corn kernels
¼ teaspoon paprika
1 tablespoon chopped cilantro or parsley
Juice of 1 lime
2 avocados, halved and pitted (peel on)
½ cup low-fat feta cheese, crumbled

1. Rinse the quinoa well to clean it, and pick out debris (if any). Pour the oil in a small sauté pan over medium heat, toast the quinoa for 1 minute. Add the water and bring just to a boil. Stir once, reduce the heat, cover, and simmer for 15 minutes. Remove from heat and fluff with a fork.

2. In a small bowl, mix the vegetables, paprika, cilantro, and lime juice. Carefully scoop some of the avocado flesh out of the peel, leaving some of the green fruit on the sides and the bottom. Chop the scooped-out avocado and add it to the vegetables, along with the feta crumbles and cooked quinoa. Fold in carefully.

3. Divide the mixture evenly and fill the avocado halves.

CALORIES **274**
TOTAL FAT **16 G**
CHOLESTEROL **0 MG**
SATURATED FAT **2 G**
TOTAL CARBOHYDRATES **31 G**

FIBER **10 G**
SUGAR **3 G**
SODIUM **11 MG**
PROTEIN **6 G**

Stacked Eggplant Caponata with Spinach and Mozzarella

SERVES 6

PREPARATION TIME **20 TO 30 MINUTES**
COOKING TIME **40 MINUTES**
TOTAL TIME **1 HOUR TO 1 HOUR 10 MINUTES**

Eggplant caponata has a wonderful sweet and sour flavor and is generally eaten as a condiment or an appetizer served on bread or crackers. Here we've used the appetizer as an inspiration to create a vegetarian entrée, made into a meal with the addition of spinach and mozzarella.

2 tablespoons extra-virgin olive oil
1 tablespoon sugar or sugar substitute
2 teaspoons Italian seasoning
2 garlic cloves, minced
¼ cup capers
¼ cup green olives, chopped
¼ cup toasted pine nuts or chopped toasted walnuts
½ cup currants or raisins
Fine-grained kosher salt and freshly ground black pepper, to taste
Olive oil cooking spray
1 large eggplant (about 1 pound), sliced into ½-inch-thick rounds
1 medium to large tomato, sliced into about ¼-inch rounds
8 ounces (about 2 cups) part skim or low-fat mozzarella cheese, cut in ¼-inch-thick slices
1 (10-ounce) package baby spinach leaves

1. Preheat the oven to 375 degrees F.

2. In a small bowl, mix together the oil, sweetener, Italian seasoning, garlic, capers, olives, nuts, and currants or raisins. Season with salt and pepper.

3. Coat one large baking pan or individual-size baking dishes or ramekins with cooking spray.

4. Layer the ingredients, starting with the eggplant, followed by the sweet-and-sour mixture, tomatoes, mozzarella, another spoonful of the sweet-and-sour mixture, spinach, and another layer of eggplant. Repeat the stacking until all the vegetables are incorporated, and pour any remaining sauce over the top.

5. Cover the pan or ramekins tightly with aluminum foil and bake for 30 minutes. Remove foil and bake for an additional 10 minutes. Let rest for 5 minutes and serve while still hot.

6. If baking in a pan, simply cut the caponata into squares and remove carefully with a spatula. If baking in individual baking dishes or ramekins, loosen the sides with a butter knife and carefully overturn the dish to gently place the stacked caponata onto a plate.

CALORIES **288**

TOTAL FAT **20 G**

CHOLESTEROL **24 MG**

SATURATED FAT **5 G**

TOTAL CARBOHYDRATES **17 G**

FIBER **8 G**

SUGAR **5 G**

SODIUM **183 MG**

PROTEIN **16 G**

Oven-Baked Eggplant Parmesan

SERVES 6

PREPARATION TIME **15 MINUTES**
COOKING TIME **55 MINUTES TO 1 HOUR 5 MINUTES**
TOTAL TIME **1 HOUR 10 MINUTES TO 1 HOUR 20 MINUTES**

Skip the frying and save fat and calories! If you bake the breaded eggplant before adding the sauce and mozzarella, you'll still have the crispy crust we all love.

Olive oil cooking spray
¾ cup plain bread crumbs
¾ cup grated Parmesan, divided
1½ teaspoons Italian seasoning
Fine-grained kosher salt and freshly ground black pepper, to taste
2 large eggplants, sliced into ½-inch-thick rounds
4 egg whites or ½ cup egg substitute
6 cups homemade or packaged low-sodium or salt-free tomato
    sauce, divided
1 cup shredded part-skim mozzarella, divided

1. Preheat the oven to 375 degrees F.

2. Coat 2 baking sheets with olive oil cooking spray. Combine the bread crumbs, ½ cup of the Parmesan, and the Italian seasoning, and season with salt and pepper.

3. Dip the eggplant slices in the egg whites. Dredge the eggplant in the bread-crumb mixture, coating well. Place the eggplant on baking sheets, and bake until crisp on bottom, about 20 to 25 minutes. Flip and bake for 20 to 25 minutes more, or until golden brown and crispy.

4. Pour 2 cups of the tomato sauce into the bottom of a large baking dish. Top with half the eggplant rounds. Cover with 2 more cups sauce and half of the mozzarella. Repeat with another layer of eggplant, the remaining sauce, and the remaining mozzarella. Sprinkle with remaining ¼ cup of Parmesan cheese.

5. Bake uncovered for 15 minutes, or until the cheese is golden and the sauce is bubbling.

CALORIES **273**

TOTAL FAT **8 G**

CHOLESTEROL **21 MG**

SATURATED FAT **4 G**

TOTAL CARBOHYDRATES **35 G**

FIBER **10 G**

SUGAR **15 G**

SODIUM **201 MG**

PROTEIN **19 G**

Kasha and Cranberry-Stuffed Acorn Squash

SERVES 4

PREPARATION TIME **10 MINUTES**
COOKING TIME **1 HOUR 10 MINUTES TO 1 HOUR 25 MINUTES**
TOTAL TIME **1 HOUR 20 MINUTES TO 1 HOUR 35 MINUTES**

This is a naturally sweet and filling dish. Serve it with your favorite greens, sautéed in a bit of olive oil and garlic, or a nice side salad, to turn it into a balanced vegetarian meal.

2 acorn squash
2 tablespoons olive oil, divided
Fine-grained kosher salt and freshly ground black pepper, to taste
1 cup buckwheat groats (kasha)
2 cups cold water
½ cup dried cranberries or raisins
Juice of 1 orange
Zest of ½ orange
Pinch of grated nutmeg
⅛ teaspoon cinnamon

1. Preheat the oven to 400 degrees F.

2. Cut the acorn squash in half, and scoop out the seeds. Place each half in a baking pan, cut side up. Add ¼ inch of water to the bottom of the pan so that the squash doesn't get dried out.

3. Drizzle ½ tablespoon of olive oil into each squash half, and season with salt and pepper. Bake for 1 hour to 1 hour 15 minutes, or until the squash is very soft and the tops are browned. Be careful not to undercook. Remove the squash from the oven, and let it cool in the pan for 10 minutes.

4. While the squash is baking, prepare the kasha. Combine the buckwheat and water in a medium-size pot, and bring to a boil over high heat. Stir and reduce the heat to simmer uncovered for 15 to 20 minutes, or until tender yet still chewy. Drain any excess water from the kasha.

5. Add the cranberries or raisins, remaining olive oil, orange juice and zest, nutmeg, and cinnamon. Stir to combine and season with more salt and pepper to taste, if desired.

6. Divide the kasha mixture, and place an equal amount into the center of each squash. Cut each one in half to serve.

CALORIES **223**

TOTAL FAT **8 G**

CHOLESTEROL **0 MG**

SATURATED FAT **1 G**

TOTAL CARBOHYDRATES **40 G**

FIBER **5 G**

SUGAR **12 G**

SODIUM **217 MG**

PROTEIN **2 G**

Stuffed Portobello Mushrooms

SERVES 4 (1 STUFFED MUSHROOM PER SERVING)

PREPARATION TIME **15 MINUTES**
COOKING TIME **50 MINUTES TO 1 HOUR**
TOTAL TIME **1 HOUR 5 MINUTES TO 1 HOUR 15 MINUTES**

Portobellos are a "meaty" mushroom and often are used as a meat substitute because they are so hearty and have such a firm texture. This Italian-inspired recipe makes them into an entrée by stuffing them.

If you don't have Italian seasoning handy, use a combination of dried basil, dried rosemary, and dried oregano.

4 large portobello mushrooms
2 tablespoons olive oil, divided
1 tablespoon balsamic vinegar
2 teaspoons Italian seasoning
1 large red onion, diced
1 medium zucchini, diced
1 roasted red pepper, seeded and diced
2 to 3 garlic cloves, minced
2 cups baby spinach
¼ cup bread crumbs
2 tablespoons chopped parsley
⅛ teaspoon crushed red pepper flakes
¼ cup freshly grated Parmesan
Fine-grained kosher salt and freshly ground black pepper, to taste
¼ cup part-skim or low-fat mozzarella cheese

1. Preheat the oven to 375 degrees F.

2. Clean the portobellos by wiping with a damp towel, remove the stems, and scrape off the brown gills with the side of a spoon. Coat the mushrooms entirely with 1 tablespoon olive oil, vinegar, and Italian seasoning.

3. In a sauté pan over medium-high heat, cook the onion in the rest of the oil until softened and translucent (about 5 minutes). Add the zucchini and continue to cook until the zucchini begins to lose some its water and soften. Add in the pepper and cook for an additional 3 minutes. Add the garlic and cook for an additional 30 seconds, until it is golden and fragrant. Add the baby spinach, stir it until just wilted, and remove it from the heat.

4. Stir in the bread crumbs, parsley, red pepper flakes, Parmesan, and season with salt and pepper. Stir well to combine. Place ¼ of the mixture inside each mushroom cap.

5. Bake for 30 to 35 minutes. Top each with equal amounts of mozzarella, and bake for a few more minutes, until the cheese is melted.

CALORIES **216**

TOTAL FAT **12 G**

CHOLESTEROL **11 MG**

SATURATED FAT **3 G**

TOTAL CARBOHYDRATES **20 G**

FIBER **4 G**

SUGAR **8 G**

SODIUM **170 MG**

PROTEIN **10 G**

Vegetable Stir-Fry

SERVES 4

PREPARATION TIME **25 MINUTES**
COOKING TIME **8 MINUTES**
TOTAL TIME **33 MINUTES**

Tofu is high in protein and is the perfect substitute for meat in any vegetarian recipe. But if you are not a fan, it can be left out of this colorful and tasty stir-fry. The key to making a good stir-fry is to heat the pan to a very high temperature so that the vegetables cook quickly and do not get mushy.

This stir-fry is traditionally served over brown rice. Other nutritious options are couscous or quinoa.

2 tablespoons canola oil
1 teaspoon ground ginger, or 1 tablespoon peeled and minced
   fresh ginger
1 red bell pepper, cored, seeded, and sliced into thin strips
1 yellow bell pepper, cored, seeded, and sliced into thin strips
1 red onion, cut in half and sliced into thin strips
1 cup broccoli florets, chopped small
½ cup snow peas or sugar snap peas
8 ounces firm tofu, chopped into bite-size pieces
¼ cup low-sodium soy sauce
2 cups chopped bok choy, Swiss chard, or spinach
Pinch of cayenne pepper
1 tablespoon sesame oil (toasted or regular)
1 clove garlic, minced
1 cup bean sprouts (optional)

1. In a wok or large skillet, heat the canola oil over high heat until shimmering. If using a wok, allow it to heat for 1 minute before adding the oil. If the oil starts smoking, turn down the heat until it stops.

2. Add the ginger, peppers, and onion, and stir constantly for 2 minutes. Add the broccoli, snow or snap peas, tofu, and soy sauce, and stir constantly for 4 to 5 minutes.

3. Add in the greens, cayenne pepper, and sesame oil, and stir for about 2 minutes, or until the greens have just wilted. Add in the minced garlic and cook for an additional 30 seconds until golden and fragrant. If using bean sprouts, stir them in now and then remove the wok or skillet from heat and serve.

CALORIES **229**

TOTAL FAT **13 G**

CHOLESTEROL **0 MG**

SATURATED FAT **2 G**

TOTAL CARBOHYDRATES **13 G**

FIBER **4 G**

SUGAR **5 G**

SODIUM **199 MG**

PROTEIN **9 G**

Vegetable Coconut Curry

SERVES 4

PREPARATION TIME **15 MINUTES**
COOKING TIME **35 TO 40 MINUTES**
TOTAL TIME **50 TO 55 MINUTES**

This recipe calls for yellow or red curry powder. If you are unfamiliar with curry powder, these are different blends of spices. Yellow curry powder has more turmeric and produces a mild-tasting dish, while the red curry powder gets its color from chili peppers and creates a spicier dish. Try a variety of curry powders until you find the flavor you like.

Serve this curry over brown basmati rice or brown rice.

1 tablespoons canola or olive oil
½ medium to large white onion, finely chopped
1-inch fresh gingerroot, peeled and finely grated
½ tablespoon ground coriander
1 tablespoon red or yellow curry powder
Pinch of cayenne pepper
½ tablespoon tomato paste
2 garlic cloves, minced
½ cup light coconut milk
1 cup homemade or commercial low-sodium vegetable stock
¼ teaspoon ground cinnamon
1 cup peeled sweet potatoes, 1-inch pieces
1 medium carrot, peeled and coarsely chopped
1 medium tomato, coarsely chopped
2 cups small cauliflower florets
1 cup canned garbanzo beans (chickpeas), rinsed and drained
4 loosely packed cups baby spinach
Juice of 1 lime
Fine-grained kosher salt, to taste
Chopped cilantro for garnish

1. In a heavy-bottomed pot, heat the oil and onion over medium heat until the onion becomes soft and translucent around the edges.

2. Add the ginger, coriander, curry powder, and cayenne, stirring to form a paste. Add the tomato paste and garlic. Allow to cook for 1 minute.

3. Add the coconut milk, stock, cinnamon, sweet potatoes, and carrot, and bring just to a boil over high heat. Reduce heat and simmer for about 10 minutes. Then add the tomato and cauliflower, and continue to simmer until the vegetables are tender, 10 to 15 more minutes.

4. Stir in the garbanzo beans, spinach, and lime juice, and cook until the spinach has wilted, about 3 minutes. Season with salt. Serve garnished with cilantro.

CALORIES **288**

TOTAL FAT **12 G**

CHOLESTEROL **1 MG**

SATURATED FAT **6 G**

TOTAL CARBOHYDRATES **41 G**

FIBER **9 G**

SUGAR **7 G**

SODIUM **155 MG**

PROTEIN **9 G**

Creamy Butternut Squash Lasagna

SERVES 8

PREPARATION TIME **20 MINUTES**
COOKING TIME **1 HOUR**
TOTAL TIME **1 HOUR 20 MINUTES**

This creamy and delicious lasagna stuffed with ricotta and butternut squash is a perfect meal on a cold day. Serve it with a side salad for a balanced and healthful meal.

1 large butternut squash, peeled, seeded, and chopped
2 tablespoons olive oil
Pinch of freshly grated nutmeg or ground nutmeg
Fine-grained kosher salt and freshly ground black pepper, to taste
2 cups part-skim ricotta cheese
2 egg whites or ¼ cup egg substitute
1 teaspoon dried sage
1 cup grated Parmesan, divided
2 cups shredded part-skim or nonfat mozzarella cheese, divided
12 whole-wheat lasagna noodles, no-boil or boiled according
    to package directions

1. Preheat the oven to 400 degrees F.

2. In a large bowl, toss the chopped squash with olive oil and nutmeg, and season with salt and pepper. Spread the squash evenly on a nonstick or parchment-lined baking sheet, and bake for 25 to 30 minutes until soft all the way through. Remove from the oven, and reduce the temperature to 375 degrees F.

3. Purée the squash in batches in a blender or food processor, adding a small amount of water, about ¼ cup in total. Note that more water can be added if necessary to achieve a smooth applesauce consistency in the squash purée. Set aside.

4. In a small bowl, combine the ricotta cheese, egg whites or substitute, sage, half of the Parmesan, and ½ cup of the mozzarella, and season with more salt and pepper, if desired. Set aside.

5. Spray a 9 × 13–inch baking pan with oil. Build the lasagna by spreading one-third of the squash purée over the bottom of the pan, cover with a layer of lasagna noodles (edges can overlap slightly), spread some of the ricotta mixture, add another layer of noodles, add the squash purée, sprinkle with some of the mozzarella, and add another layer of noodles. Repeat the layering, ending with a layer of noodles. Sprinkle the remaining mozzarella and Parmesan over the top.

6. Spray a piece of aluminum foil with nonstick spray (so the cheese doesn't stick) and cover the pan. Bake for 30 minutes, remove the foil, and bake for 5 minutes more, or until heated through.

CALORIES **284**

TOTAL FAT **16 G**

CHOLESTEROL **46 MG**

SATURATED FAT **9 G**

TOTAL CARBOHYDRATES **15 G**

FIBER **2 G**

SUGAR **3 G**

SODIUM **174 MG**

PROTEIN **20 G**

Southwest Stuffed Red Bell Peppers

SERVES 6 (½ A PEPPER PER SERVING)

PREPARATION TIME **15 MINUTES**
COOKING TIME **40 TO 45 MINUTES**
TOTAL TIME **55 MINUTES TO 1 HOUR**

This recipe is a fun take on stuffed peppers. What could be better than a meal of chili and rice in a bell pepper package smothered with cheese? It's truly a fiesta of flavor.

½ medium white onion, chopped
½ medium jalapeño, seeded and minced (optional)
1 tablespoon olive oil
1 garlic clove, minced
1¼ cups cooked brown rice, instant or regular
¾ cup canned black beans, rinsed and drained
¾ cup frozen or fresh corn kernels
½ cup low-sodium or no-salt-added canned tomato sauce or purée
1 teaspoon chili powder
½ teaspoon ground cumin
Fine-grained kosher salt and freshly ground black pepper, to taste
3 medium-size red bell peppers, cored, seeded, and halved
1 tablespoon chopped cilantro
¾ cup shredded reduced-fat cheddar cheese

1. Preheat the oven to 375 degrees F.

2. Heat the onion and jalapeño, if using, in oil over medium heat until the onion has softened and is translucent at the edges. Cook the garlic in oil for 30 seconds until golden and fragrant. Add in the cooked rice, beans, corn, tomato sauce, chili powder, and cumin, and stir well. Season with salt and pepper, and remove from heat.

3. Divide the mixture evenly and fill each of the pepper halves. Arrange peppers in a 9 × 13–inch baking dish that has been sprayed with nonstick spray, and bake for 25 to 30 minutes or until the peppers are soft. Sprinkle with cilantro and cheese, and bake for 5 more minutes, or until the cheese is melted.

CALORIES **216**

TOTAL FAT **8 G**

CHOLESTEROL **16 MG**

SATURATED FAT **4 G**

TOTAL CARBOHYDRATES **28 G**

FIBER **6 G**

SUGAR **4 G**

SODIUM **175 MG**

PROTEIN **9 G**

Bursting Burritos with Tofu and Black Beans

SERVES 4

PREPARATION TIME **20 MINUTES**
COOKING TIME **10 MINUTES**
TOTAL TIME **30 MINUTES**

A complete meal in a wrap! You'll love these zesty burritos; they are not only filling and tasty, they are fun to make and eat. Instead of taco night, try this healthful alternative.

1 tablespoon olive oil
½ cup chopped red onion
½ teaspoon ground cumin
¼ teaspoon ground turmeric (optional)
1 cup firm tofu, crumbled
1 cup cored, seeded, and chopped red or yellow bell pepper
1 jalapeño, seeded and minced (optional)
1 cup canned black beans, rinsed and drained
1 garlic clove, minced
½ cup grated reduced-fat cheddar cheese
1 cup chopped tomatoes
1 avocado, peeled, pitted, and chopped
Fine-grained kosher salt and freshly ground black pepper, to taste
4 large whole-wheat tortillas or wraps
2 tablespoons chopped cilantro

1. Preheat the oven to 350 degrees F.

2. Heat the oil in large nonstick skillet over medium-high heat. Add the onion and cook over medium heat until it is softened and translucent at the edges. Add the cumin and turmeric, and stir for 30 seconds. Add the tofu, bell peppers, jalapeño (if using), and black beans, and cook until heated through. Add the garlic and cook for about 30 seconds. Add the cheddar cheese and remove from the heat. Stir in the tomatoes and avocado. Season with salt and pepper.

3. Add the filling to the center of each wrap, top with some of the cilantro, and fold into a burrito. Serve immediately.

CALORIES **524**

TOTAL FAT **24 G**

CHOLESTEROL **13 MG**

SATURATED FAT **6 G**

TOTAL CARBOHYDRATES **60 G**

FIBER **10 G**

SUGAR **4 G**

SODIUM **155 MG**

PROTEIN **21 G**

Pastas

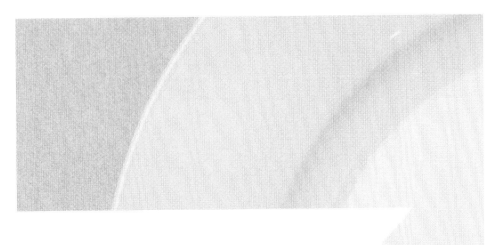

CHAPTER TEN

Pastas

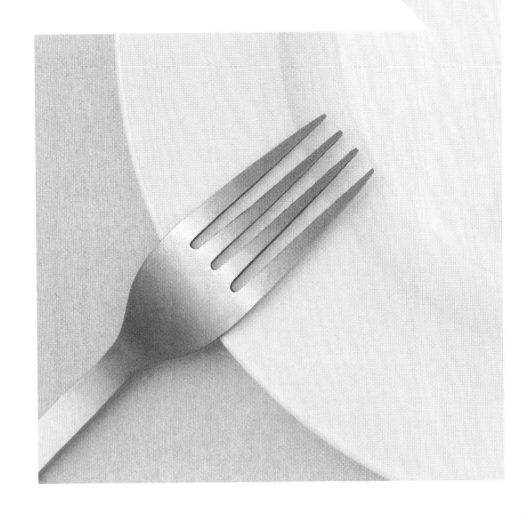

Fettuccine with Pink Sauce

PREPARATION TIME **5 MINUTES**
COOKING TIME **30 TO 35 MINUTES (PLUS TIME TO COOK THE PASTA)**
TOTAL TIME **35 TO 40 MINUTES (PLUS TIME TO COOK THE PASTA)**

You're in for a treat if you've never tried pink sauce, and this creamy version is absolutely perfect for fettuccine. The trick to a light but creamy sauce is combining nonfat milk with cornstarch instead of using fat- and calorie-laden heavy cream.

8 ounces uncooked egg fettuccine
2 tablespoons extra-virgin olive oil
½ medium onion, finely chopped
2 garlic cloves, minced
1 (15-ounce) can low-sodium or salt-free tomato sauce or
    marinara sauce
1 teaspoon granulated sweetener or equivalent
Fine-grained kosher salt and freshly ground black pepper, to taste
½ cup nonfat evaporated milk plus 1 teaspoon cornstarch, whisked
    to form a slurry
¼ cup grated Parmesan cheese
Chopped fresh basil for garnish

1. Cook the pasta according to the package directions, drain (reserving ½ cup of the cooking water), rinse so that the fettuccine doesn't stick together, and return it to the cooking pot. Set aside.

2. Add the olive oil and onion to a large skillet over medium heat and cook for about 5 minutes, until the onion has softened and is translucent. Add the garlic and cook for an additional 30 seconds. Pour in the tomato sauce and add the sweetener, then season with salt and pepper. Cook over low heat for 25 to 30 minutes, stirring occasionally.

continued ▶

3. Remove from the heat, and stir in the milk slurry and Parmesan cheese. Add enough of the reserved cooking water to loosen the sauce so it appears creamy. Pour the sauce over the pasta, toss to coat, pour the pasta into a serving dish. Garnish with basil before serving.

CALORIES **335**

TOTAL FAT **11 G**

CHOLESTEROL **7 MG**

SATURATED FAT **2 G**

TOTAL CARBOHYDRATES **54 G**

FIBER **8 G**

SUGAR **6 G**

SODIUM **677 MG**

PROTEIN **9 G**

Macaroni and Cheese

SERVES 4

PREPARATION TIME **5 MINUTES (PLUS TIME TO COOK THE PASTA)**
COOKING TIME **15 TO 20 MINUTES**
TOTAL TIME **20 TO 25 MINUTES (PLUS TIME TO COOK THE PASTA)**

No matter what your age is, macaroni and cheese is a great comfort food. This velvety, light version is made with a creamy sauce and topped with panko bread crumbs and a sprinkle of cheddar for extra-crispy deliciousness. Panko are larger than regular bread crumbs, so use them for an added crunch. You can find them at most grocery stores.

Serve the mac and cheese with a side of green vegetables such as broccoli or spinach, or a side salad with leafy greens.

Olive oil cooking spray
2 cups (8 ounces) dry whole-wheat elbow pasta, cooked
    according to package directions and drained
¾ cup panko (Japanese-style) or plain bread crumbs
4½ teaspoons olive oil, divided
¼ teaspoon salt, divided
Freshly ground black pepper, to taste
1 tablespoon all-purpose flour
1 cup 1 percent low-fat milk
⅛ teaspoon ground or freshly grated nutmeg
¾ cup reduced-fat cheddar cheese, divided

1. Preheat the oven to 350 degrees F. Spray a 13 × 9–inch baking pan with cooking spray.

2. In a small bowl, combine the bread crumbs with the 1½ teaspoons of the olive oil, ⅛ teaspoon of the salt, and season with pepper. Set aside.

3. In a large saucepan, over medium heat, whisk the rest of the olive oil and flour constantly until it forms a roux and turns a golden hue and has a nutty fragrance (3 to 5 minutes). Do not stop whisking, or the roux will burn.

continued ▶

4. With the heat still on medium, slowly drizzle in the milk, whisking constantly and briskly the whole time. Stir until the sauce becomes the consistency of very thick cream. Whisk in the nutmeg. Remove from the heat, and whisk in ¼ cup of the grated cheddar until melted and fully combined with the sauce. Add the pasta and stir well to coat.

5. Pour the cheesy noodles into the prepared baking pan, and cover with a layer of the remaining cheddar and then top with the bread-crumb mixture. Bake uncovered for 10 to 15 minutes, or until the bread crumbs are golden and the cheese has melted.

CALORIES **461**

TOTAL FAT **17 G**

CHOLESTEROL **30 MG**

SATURATED FAT **7 G**

TOTAL CARBOHYDRATES **62 G**

FIBER **7 G**

SUGAR **1 G**

SODIUM **157 MG**

PROTEIN **16 G**

Shrimp Lo Mein

SERVES 4

PREPARATION TIME **20 MINUTES (PLUS TIME TO COOK THE PASTA OR NOODLES)**
COOKING TIME **10 MINUTES**
TOTAL TIME **30 MINUTES (PLUS TIME TO COOK THE PASTA OR NOODLES)**

When you've got a craving for lo mein, try making this easy and healthier version at home. This recipe calls for oyster sauce or hoisin (a sweet barbecue sauce), but if you can't find either in the Asian food section of your supermarket, then substitute Worcestershire sauce. You'll also need a chili paste, such as sriracha or sambal oelek. If you don't have any, use crushed pepper flakes.

Also note that any of the three types of cabbage can be used. Both napa and savoy have softer leaves, while green cabbage adds crunch. Make sure you shred the cabbage as thinly as possible, as with coleslaw.

8 ounces dry whole-wheat thin spaghetti or Chinese egg noodles
1 tablespoon canola oil, divided
2 cups (½ pound) snow peas or sugar snap peas
1 pound small uncooked shrimp, peeled and deveined
2 stalks celery, very thinly sliced
½ cup red or yellow bell pepper, cored, seeded, and sliced into strips
1-inch piece gingerroot, peeled and grated
1 cup finely shredded napa cabbage, savoy cabbage, or
    green cabbage
5 scallions, white and green parts divided, thinly sliced
2 garlic cloves, minced
¼ cup cold water
¼ cup oyster sauce or ⅛ cup hoisin sauce or 2 tablespoons
    Worcestershire sauce
½ tablespoon sesame oil (toasted or regular)
2 tablespoons rice vinegar or apple cider vinegar
½ teaspoon equivalent measure sugar substitute
1 tablespoon low-sodium soy sauce
Sriracha hot sauce, sambal oelek, or crushed red peppers, to taste

continued ▶

1. Cook the noodles according to the package directions. Drain well and toss with a tiny bit of oil to keep from sticking and set aside.

2. Remove the strings from the sugar snap peas or snow peas by snapping off the stem end and pulling the string downward along the length of the pod.

3. Heat the rest of the oil in a wok or large skillet over high heat. If using a wok, heat the wok for 1 minute before adding the oil. Stir-fry the shrimp for 2 to 3 minutes, until they're pink and cooked through. Remove with a slotted spoon. Add the celery, bell pepper, and ginger, and cook for 2 minutes; then add the cabbage, peas, scallion whites, and garlic. Stir to combine and cook through, about 2 to 3 more minutes.

4. Add the water, oyster sauce (or hoisin or Worcestershire), sesame oil, vinegar, sweetener, and soy sauce. Stir and cook until the sauce thickens, about 1 to 2 minutes. Add the shrimp and noodles, and stir to combine.

5. Serve with hot sauce or crushed red peppers on the side.

174

CALORIES **357**

TOTAL FAT **8 G**

CHOLESTEROL **143 MG**

SATURATED FAT **1 G**

TOTAL CARBOHYDRATES **52 G**

FIBER **8 G**

SUGAR **2 G**

SODIUM **270 MG**

PROTEIN **21 G**

The Diabetic Cookbook

Turkey and Spinach Lasagna

SERVES 8

PREPARATION TIME **5 MINUTES**
COOKING TIME **1 HOUR**
TOTAL TIME **1 HOUR 5 MINUTES**

A ground turkey Bolognese sauce, three cheeses, and wilted spinach create this lovely creamy and satisfying lasagna. Serve with a crisp green salad and you've got the perfect meal.

2 tablespoons extra-virgin olive oil, divided
1 medium onion, finely chopped
3 garlic cloves, minced
1 (10 ounce) package baby spinach
1 pound ground turkey
1 (28-ounce) can crushed tomatoes
1 (6-ounce) can tomato paste
1 tablespoon Italian seasoning
15 ounces part-skim ricotta cheese
2 cups (8 ounces) part-skim shredded mozzarella cheese, divided
¾ cup freshly grated Parmesan cheese, divided
2 egg whites or ¼ cup egg substitute
½ teaspoon salt
Freshly ground black pepper, to taste
1 (8-ounce) package whole-wheat lasagna noodles (no-boil
    or precooked)

1. Preheat the oven to 400 degrees F.

2. Add 1 tablespoon of olive oil and the onion to a large skillet over medium heat and cook for about 5 minutes, until softened and translucent. Add the garlic and cook for 30 seconds more, until just golden and fragrant. Add the baby spinach and 1 tablespoon of water and cook until just wilted. Cover the pan if necessary to steam. Remove the spinach to a bowl and set aside.

continued ▶

3. Use the same pan to saute the ground turkey over medium heat until it is no longer pink, about 10 minutes. Add the crushed tomatoes, tomato paste, and Italian seasoning, and salt, season with pepper, then simmer uncovered for about 20 minutes, stirring occasionally.

4. In a large bowl, combine the ricotta, ½ cup of mozzarella, half the Parmesan cheese, and eggs, and stir until well combined.

5. Coat a 13 × 19–inch baking pan with cooking spray. Spoon a layer of turkey sauce into the bottom of the pan. Cover with a layer of lasagna noodles and top with one-third of the ricotta mixture and one-third of the wilted spinach. Add another layer of noodles and repeat process two more times, ending with a layer of lasagna noodles topped with 1 tablespoon of olive oil.

6. Sprinkle the remaining Parmesan over the top. Coat one side of aluminum foil with nonstick cooking spray, and place spray-side down and covering lasagna tightly. Bake for 20 minutes or until tomato sauce is bubbling. Uncover and bake for an additional 5 minutes. Remove the lasagna from the oven, and let it rest for 5 minutes before cutting into 8 portions. Serve hot.

CALORIES **471**
TOTAL FAT **21 G**
CHOLESTEROL **92 MG**
SATURATED FAT **10 G**
TOTAL CARBOHYDRATES **39 G**

FIBER **6 G**
SUGAR **7 G**
SODIUM **191 MG**
PROTEIN **34 G**

Fettuccine Alfredo with Broccoli

SERVES 4

PREPARATION TIME **5 MINUTES (PLUS TIME TO COOK THE PASTA AND STEAM THE BROCCOLI)**
COOKING TIME **5 TO 10 MINUTES**
TOTAL TIME **10 TO 15 MINUTES (PLUS TIME TO COOK THE PASTA AND STEAM THE BROCCOLI)**

Fettuccine is a hearty noodle, and together with the added broccoli makes for a substantial serving size of two cups. The broccoli increases the nutritional value with its powerhouse of nutrients and tastes great with fettuccine.

1 cup 1 percent milk
6 whole garlic cloves, peeled
1 teaspoon lemon zest
⅛ teaspoon ground or freshly grated nutmeg
¼ tablespoon fine-grained kosher salt
Freshly ground black pepper, to taste
2 tablespoons nonfat cream cheese
¾ cup grated Parmesan cheese
3 tablespoons chopped fresh parsley
8 ounces egg fettuccine noodles, cooked according to package directions, ½ cup cooking water reserved
4 heaping cups raw broccoli florets, steamed and drained

1. In a small saucepan, combine the milk, garlic, lemon zest, nutmeg, and salt, and season with pepper. Simmer the mixture uncovered over medium heat until the garlic has softened and the milk has reduced or thickened.

continued ▶

2. Purée the hot garlic and milk mixture in the pot with an immersion blender or in a standing blender, holding down the lid with a kitchen towel while puréeing. Whisk in the cream cheese and the Parmesan until fully incorporated. If the sauce does not appear creamy, add any of the reserved cooking water to loosen it up. Add the parsley.

3. Pour the sauce over the noodles, add the broccoli, and toss to combine.

CALORIES **392**

TOTAL FAT **11 G**

CHOLESTEROL **31 MG**

SATURATED FAT **6 G**

TOTAL CARBOHYDRATES **57 G**

FIBER **9 G**

SUGAR **5 G**

SODIUM **124 MG**

PROTEIN **18 G**

Spaghetti Bolognese

SERVES 4

PREPARATION TIME **10 MINUTES (PLUS TIME TO COOK THE PASTA)**
COOKING TIME **30 MINUTES**
TOTAL TIME **40 MINUTES (PLUS TIME TO COOK THE PASTA)**

When you crave spaghetti with meat sauce, make this healthier version of the classic. Traditional Bolognese is made with pork and beef, but try using turkey for a leaner, less greasy result. This spaghetti is so filling and delicious that you'll be more than satisfied with the taste and the portion.

2 tablespoons extra-virgin olive oil
1 medium onion, chopped
1 large carrot, peeled and chopped
2 stalks celery chopped
2 garlic cloves, minced
1 pound lean ground turkey or 85 percent lean ground beef
½ teaspoon fine-grained kosher salt, divided
Freshly ground black pepper, to taste
1 tablespoon Italian seasoning
½ cup red wine or ½ cup low-sodium beef stock
½ cup tomato paste
1½ cups low-sodium tomato sauce or purée
8 ounces whole-wheat spaghetti of choice, cooked according to
    package directions
¼ cup grated Parmesan

1. Heat the olive oil in a sauté pan or skillet, and add the onion, carrot, and celery, and cook until the onion is translucent and softened. Add in the garlic and cook for 30 seconds until the garlic is golden and fragrant.

continued ▶

2. Stir in the raw meat and half the salt, and season with pepper. Add Italian seasoning, and cook for 10 minutes over medium heat or until well browned. Add the wine or stock and the tomato paste, and cook for an additional 5 minutes, until some of the liquid has evaporated. Add the tomato sauce and the remaining salt, and simmer on low heat for 10 minutes longer.

3. Pour the sauce over the pasta, toss to combine, and serve immediately with the grated Parmesan.

CALORIES **338**

TOTAL FAT **17 G**

CHOLESTEROL **103 MG**

SATURATED FAT **5 G**

TOTAL CARBOHYDRATES **19 G**

FIBER **4 G**

SUGAR **11 G**

SODIUM **208 MG**

PROTEIN **26 G**

Pasta Primavera

SERVES 4

PREPARATION TIME **15 TO 20 MINUTES (PLUS TIME TO COOK
    THE PASTA)**
COOKING TIME **10 MINUTES**
TOTAL TIME **25 TO 30 MINUTES (PLUS TIME TO COOK THE PASTA)**

*Pasta primavera is such a versatile dish because you can substitute your favor-
ite nonstarchy vegetables, depending on the season, what you've picked up at
the farmer's market, or what's in the refrigerator. What's more, it's a great way
to enjoy pasta without loading up on carbs.*

2 tablespoons extra-virgin olive oil
2 medium carrots, peeled and finely chopped
1 medium onion, finely chopped
1 small zucchini, diced
1 medium yellow, red, or green bell pepper, cored, seeded, and
    finely chopped
½ cup frozen peas, thawed
1½ cups halved cherry tomatoes
¼ teaspoon salt
Freshly ground black pepper, to taste
3 garlic cloves, minced
¼ cup grated Parmesan
8 ounces whole-wheat penne, farfalle, or ziti pasta, cooked accord-
    ing to package directions, ½ cup cooking water reserved
Chopped basil for garnish

1. Heat the olive oil in a large sauté pan or skillet over medium heat. Add the
carrots and cook for 3 minutes. Add the onion, zucchini, and bell pepper,
and cook for an additional 3 to 5 minutes until softened. Add the peas and
tomatoes, and cook for 2 minutes. Season with salt and pepper, and stir. Add
the garlic and cook for 30 seconds until the garlic is golden and fragrant.

continued ▶

2. Toss the pasta with the Parmesan and the reserved pasta water. Toss in the vegetables and garnish with the basil.

CALORIES **344**

TOTAL FAT **11 G**

CHOLESTEROL **5 MG**

SATURATED FAT **2 G**

TOTAL CARBOHYDRATES **56 G**

FIBER **9 G**

SUGAR **5 G**

SODIUM **156 MG**

PROTEIN **9 G**

Spaghetti with Roasted Squash and Sage–Butter Sauce

SERVES 4

PREPARATION TIME **5 MINUTES (PLUS TIME TO COOK THE PASTA)**
COOKING TIME **25 MINUTES**
TOTAL TIME **30 MINUTES (PLUS TIME TO COOK THE PASTA)**

This dish is traditionally served in the late fall, when the fresh vegetables of summer are gradually replaced by heartier squash and pumpkins.

4 cups peeled, seeded, and cubed butternut squash
3 tablespoons olive oil, divided
¼ teaspoon fine-grained kosher salt
Freshly ground black pepper, to taste
2 tablespoons unsalted butter
8 fresh sage leaves
Juice of ½ lemon
8 ounces whole-wheat spaghetti, cooked according to package
    directions, ½ cup cooking water reserved
¼ cup freshly grated Parmesan cheese

Pastas

1. Preheat the oven to 400 degrees F.

2. Toss the squash in 1 tablespoon of the olive oil, season with salt and pepper, and spread in an even layer on a baking sheet. Roast for 20 minutes, or until tender. Set aside.

3. Melt the butter in the rest of the olive oil, and cook over medium heat until a golden brown color is reached. Add the sage and cook for 30 seconds longer. Remove the butter mixture from the heat, and stir in the lemon juice.

4. Coat the pasta with the sage-butter sauce, sprinkle it with Parmesan, and toss it with the squash. If the sauce is not creamy, stir in up to 1/2 cup of the reserved cooking water to loosen up the sauce. Serve hot.

CALORIES **370**
TOTAL FAT **21 G**
CHOLESTEROL **22 MG**
SATURATED FAT **8 G**
TOTAL CARBOHYDRATES **41 G**

FIBER **8 G**
SUGAR **4 G**
SODIUM **191 MG**

Linguine with Red Clam Sauce

SERVES 4

PREPARATION TIME **5 MINUTES (PLUS TIME TO COOK THE PASTA)**
COOKING TIME **10 MINUTES**
TOTAL TIME **15 MINUTES (PLUS TIME TO COOK THE PASTA)**

Clams are low in fat and calories, and although this recipe can also be modified as white clam sauce, red is more popular. When using fresh clams, always make sure they do not have an odor and are closed tightly when you buy them. After cooking, toss any that have not opened.

¼ cup extra-virgin olive oil
4 garlic cloves, thinly sliced
¼ to ½ teaspoon red pepper flakes
24 Manila or littleneck clams, well scrubbed, or 15 ounces canned
    or frozen chopped clams
1 (15-ounce) can no-added-salt diced tomatoes
½ cup dry white wine or clam juice
½ cup plus 2 tablespoons coarsely chopped fresh flat-leaf parsley
8 ounces whole-wheat linguine, cooked according to package
    directions, ½ cup cooking water reserved

1. Heat the olive oil in a large skillet or sauté pan over medium heat. Add the garlic and red pepper flakes, and cook for 30 seconds, or until the garlic is golden and fragrant. Add the clams, tomatoes, and wine or clam juice, and cook for 6 to 8 minutes. If using live clams, cook just until the clams have opened (discard any unopened clams). Stir in the parsley.

2. Transfer the linguine to serving dish (use some or all of the reserved pasta water to loosen up the pasta, if needed). Top with the sauce and serve immediately.

CALORIES **291**
TOTAL FAT **18 G**
CHOLESTEROL **26 MG**
SATURATED FAT **3 G**
TOTAL CARBOHYDRATES **9 G**

FIBER **1G**
SUGAR **2 G**
SODIUM **330 MG**
PROTEIN **14 G**

Pad Thai

SERVES 4

PREPARATION TIME **15 TO 20 MINUTES (PLUS TIME TO COOK THE NOODLES)**
COOKING TIME **8 MINUTES**
TOTAL TIME **23 TO 28 MINUTES (PLUS TIME TO COOK THE NOODLES)**

This signature Thai noodle dish is incredibly popular, but the restaurant version is usually high in fat and calories. Tamarind paste and fish sauce are what give Pad Thai its signature sweet-and-sour flavor, but substitutions are provided in the recipe if you don't have these ingredients handy.

Depending on your personal preference, you can use chicken, shrimp, or tofu, or a combination, as the protein.

¾ tablespoons tamarind paste dissolved in ¼ cup warm water or
   ¼ cup fresh lime juice mixed with 1 tablespoon brown
   sugar equivalent
2 tablespoons fish sauce or 2 teaspoons Worcestershire sauce
1 to 3 teaspoons chili sauce or ½ teaspoon red chili pepper flakes
Sweetener equivalent to 2 tablespoons brown sugar
3 scallions, white and green parts divided, sliced
1 tablespoon canola oil
4 garlic cloves, minced
1 or 2 fresh small red or green chiles such as Thai bird or serrano
   (optional), minced
3 tablespoons low-sodium soy sauce and 1 tablespoon cornstarch,
   whisked to form slurry
8 ounces Thai rice noodles, cooked according to package
   directions and rinsed in cool water to prevent sticking
1 cooked chicken breast (skin removed), sliced, or 1½ cups small
   cooked shrimp or 1½ cups finely chopped firm tofu
3 cups fresh bean sprouts
⅓ cup roughly chopped unsalted peanuts for garnish
½ cup fresh chopped cilantro for garnish

continued ▶

1. Whisk the tamarind paste, fish sauce, chili sauce, and sweetener together in a small bowl and add in the scallion whites. Set aside.

2. Add the oil to a large skillet or sauté pan and place over medium heat. Add the garlic and chiles and cook for about 30 seconds until the garlic is golden and fragrant.

3. Add the soy sauce slurry and the cooked noodles, tossing constantly for 1 minute.

4. Add the chicken, shrimp, or tofu and the tamarind sauce, and stir constantly over high heat for 3 to 5 minutes, or until all the ingredients are incorporated and heated through. Remove from the heat and toss in the bean sprouts.

5. Serve immediately, garnished with the peanuts, cilantro, and scallion greens.

CALORIES **412**

TOTAL FAT **10 G**

CHOLESTEROL **59 MG**

SATURATED FAT **1 G**

TOTAL CARBOHYDRATES **67 G**

FIBER **4 G**

SUGAR **14 G**

SODIUM **244 MG**

PROTEIN **15 G**

Tuna Noodle Casserole

SERVES 6

PREPARATION TIME **20 MINUTES (PLUS TIME TO COOK THE PASTA)**
COOKING TIME **20 TO 30 MINUTES**
TOTAL TIME **40 TO 50 MINUTES (PLUS TIME TO COOK THE PASTA)**

This tuna casserole is a classic. When you're feeling in the mood for a dish from your childhood, put this casserole together, stick it in the oven, and get ready to eat.

3 tablespoons extra-virgin olive oil, divided
2 cups sliced button mushrooms
1 tablespoon chopped fresh thyme or ½ tablespoon dried thyme
2 garlic cloves, minced
½ cup dry white wine
1 cup panko (Japanese-style) or plain bread crumbs
¼ cup freshly grated Parmesan cheese
1 tablespoon all-purpose flour
1 cup 1 percent milk, divided
⅛ teaspoon ground or freshly grated nutmeg
½ teaspoon fine-grained kosher salt
Freshly ground black pepper, to taste
1 cup frozen peas, thawed
2 (5-ounce) cans albacore tuna in water, drained and flaked
8 ounces wide egg noodles, cooked according to package directions
Chopped fresh parsley for garnish

1. Preheat the broiler on medium.

2. In the bottom of a large saucepan, over medium-high heat, heat 1 tablespoon of olive oil and add in the sliced mushrooms and thyme, cooking for 5 to 8 minutes, or until the mushrooms have released their water and it has evaporated and the mushrooms are golden. Add the garlic and cook for 30 seconds. Add the wine and cook until it has evaporated by half. Empty the contents of the pan into a bowl and set aside.

continued ▶

3. In a small bowl, mix the bread crumbs and Parmesan with 1 tablespoon of olive oil.

4. Using the large saucepan again, heat the remaining tablespoon of olive oil and whisk in the flour, stirring constantly until it reaches a golden hue and has a nutty fragrance, 3 to 5 minutes. Do not stop whisking or the paste can burn.

5. With the heat still on medium, slowly drizzle in the milk, whisking constantly and briskly. The sauce should become the consistency of very thick cream. Whisk in the nutmeg, and season with salt and pepper. Add in the mushroom mixture and the peas, and continue to whisk for about 2 minutes.

6. Remove the pan from the heat and stir in the tuna and cooked noodles. Coat a 13 x 9–baking dish with cooking spray and empty the contents into it. Top with the bread crumb mixture, and place under the broiler for 3 minutes, or until golden and crispy. Top with the fresh parsley and serve.

CALORIES **505**

TOTAL FAT **16 G**

CHOLESTEROL **58 MG**

SATURATED FAT **4 G**

TOTAL CARBOHYDRATES **57 G**

FIBER **4 G**

SUGAR **5 G**

SODIUM **279 MG**

PROTEIN **30 G**

Seafood and Poultry Dishes

Seafood and Poultry Dishes

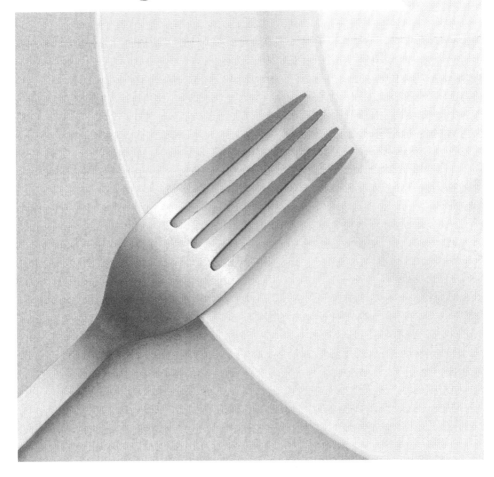

Chicken Marsala

PREPARATION TIME **5 MINUTES**
COOKING TIME **40 MINUTES**
TOTAL TIME **45 MINUTES**

The secret to this Italian classic is to pound the chicken breasts thin between two pieces of wax paper, so they cook quickly and evenly. Small servings of meat and large portions of vegetables are easy to achieve with this entrée.

¼ cup olive oil
4 boneless, skinless chicken breasts, pounded thin
Fine-grained kosher salt and freshly ground black pepper, to taste
¼ cup whole-wheat flour
½ pound mushrooms, sliced
1 cup marsala wine
1 cup chicken stock
¼ cup chopped fresh flat-leaf parsley

1. Heat the olive oil in a large skillet on medium-high heat. Season the chicken breasts with salt and pepper; then dredge them in flour. Sauté them in the olive oil until golden brown. Transfer them to an oven-safe plate, and keep warm in the oven on low.

2. Sauté the mushrooms in the same pan. Add the wine and chicken stock, and bring to a simmer. Simmer for 10 minutes, or until the sauce is reduced and thickened slightly.

3. Return the chicken to the pan, and cook it in the sauce for 10 minutes.

4. Transfer everything to a serving dish and sprinkle with the parsley.

CALORIES **437**
TOTAL FAT **11 G**
CHOLESTEROL **148 MG**
SATURATED FAT **3 G**
TOTAL CARBOHYDRATES **12 G**

FIBER **2 G**
SUGAR **1 G**
SODIUM **371 MG**
PROTEIN **57 G**

Braised Chicken with Wild Mushrooms

SERVES 4

PREPARATION TIME **15 MINUTES**
COOKING TIME **1 HOUR 45 MINUTES**
TOTAL TIME **2 HOURS**

This Italian stew is hearty and satisfying, and can be served with a variety of vegetables or salads. Stews improve with time, so make this the night before you want to serve it.

¼ cup dried porcini or morel mushrooms
¼ cup olive oil
2 or 3 slices low-salt turkey bacon, chopped
1 chicken, cut into pieces
Fine-grained kosher salt and freshly ground black pepper, to taste
1 small celery stalk, diced
1 small dried red chile, chopped
¼ cup vermouth or white wine
¼ cup tomato purée
¼ cup low-salt chicken stock
½ teaspoon arrowroot powder
¼ cup chopped fresh flat-leaf parsley
4 teaspoons fresh thyme, chopped
1 tablespoon fresh tarragon

1. Place the mushrooms in a small bowl, and pour boiling water over them. Allow them to stand for 20 minutes to soften. Strain and chop, reserving the liquid.

2. Heat the olive oil in a heavy stew pot on medium heat. Add the bacon and cook until it is browned and slightly crisp. Drain the bacon on a paper towel.

3. Season the chicken with salt and pepper, and add it to the oil and bacon drippings. Cook for 10 to 15 minutes, turning halfway through the cooking time so that both sides of the chicken are golden brown.

4. Add the celery and chopped chile, and cook for 3 to 5 minutes or until soft. Deglaze the pan with the wine, using a wooden spoon to scrape up the brown bits stuck to the bottom. Add the tomato purée, chicken stock, arrowroot powder, and mushroom liquid. Cover and simmer on low for 45 minutes.

5. Add the fresh chopped herbs and cook an additional 10 minutes, or until the sauce thickens. Season with salt and pepper.

6. Serve with wilted greens or crunchy green beans.

CALORIES **306**
TOTAL FAT **20 G**
CHOLESTEROL **71 MG**
SATURATED FAT **4 G**
TOTAL CARBOHYDRATES **6 G**

FIBER **1 G**
SUGAR **2 G**
SODIUM **173 MG**
PROTEIN **22 G**

Seafood and Poultry Dishes

Roast Chicken

SERVES 4

PREPARATION TIME **15 MINUTES**
COOKING TIME **1 HOUR 10 MINUTES TO 1 HOUR 35 MINUTES**
TOTAL TIME **1 HOUR 25 MINUTES TO 1 HOUR 50 MINUTES**

Roast chicken may seem intimidating, but it's actually one of the simplest chicken dishes you can make. Prepare this chicken for a lazy Sunday dinner, and you'll have leftovers for lunch on Monday.

¼ cup white wine
2 tablespoons olive oil, divided
1 tablespoon Dijon mustard
1 garlic clove, minced
1 teaspoon dried rosemary
Juice and zest of 1 lemon
Fine-grained kosher salt and freshly ground pepper, to taste
1 large roasting chicken, giblets removed
3 large carrots, peeled and cut into chunks
1 fennel bulb, peeled and cut into ½-inch cubes
2 celery stalks, cut into chunks

1. Preheat the oven to 400 degrees F.

2. Combine the white wine, 1 tablespoon of olive oil, mustard, garlic, rosemary, and lemon juice and zest in a bowl, and season with salt and pepper.

3. Place the chicken in a shallow roasting pan on a roasting rack. Rub the entire chicken, including the cavity, with the wine and mustard mixture. Place the chicken in the oven and roast for 15 minutes.

4. Toss the vegetables with the remaining tablespoon of olive oil, and place them around the chicken. Turn the oven temperature down to 375 degrees F. Roast an additional 40 to 60 minutes, basting the chicken every 15 minutes with the drippings in the bottom of the pan.

5. Cook the chicken until the internal temperature reaches between 170 and 180 degrees F on an instant-read thermometer inserted between the thigh and the body of the chicken. When the thermometer is removed, the juices should run clear.

6. Let the chicken rest for at least 10 to 15 minutes before serving.

CALORIES **217**

TOTAL FAT **8 G**

CHOLESTEROL **64 MG**

SATURATED FAT **6 G**

TOTAL CARBOHYDRATES **12 G**

FIBER **4 G**

SUGAR **3 G**

SODIUM **244 MG**

PROTEIN **20 G**

Seafood and Poultry Dishes

Marinated Chicken

SERVES 4

PREPARATION TIME **10 MINUTES (PLUS REFRIGERATION TIME)**
COOKING TIME **15 TO 20 MINUTES**
TOTAL TIME **25 TO 30 MINUTES (PLUS REFRIGERATION TIME)**

This Italian-inspired chicken has a bright, fresh taste from the combination of lemon and rosemary. Lean chicken breasts are a good choice for cutting calories.

½ cup olive oil
2 tablespoon fresh rosemary
1 teaspoon minced garlic
Juice and zest of 1 lemon
¼ cup chopped fresh flat-leaf parsley
Fine-grained kosher salt and freshly ground black pepper, to taste
4 boneless, skinless chicken breasts

1. Mix all the ingredients except the chicken together in a plastic bag or bowl. Place the chicken in the container, and shake or stir so the marinade thoroughly coats the chicken. Refrigerate up to 24 hours.

2. Heat a grill to medium heat and cook the chicken for 6 to 8 minutes a side. Turn only once during the cooking process.

3. Serve with a Greek salad and brown rice.

CALORIES **386**
TOTAL FAT **31 G**
CHOLESTEROL **65 MG**
SATURATED FAT **5 G**
TOTAL CARBOHYDRATES **2 G**

FIBER **1 G**
SUGAR **0 G**
SODIUM **42 MG**
PROTEIN **25 G**

Almond-Crusted Salmon

SERVES 4

PREPARATION TIME **10 MINUTES**
COOKING TIME **8 TO 12 MINUTES**
TOTAL TIME **18 TO 22 MINUTES**

Crushed almonds give this salmon a sweet and savory crunch. Salmon and almonds are both a good source of healthful fats. Make enough to use the leftovers in a green salad.

¼ cup olive oil
1 tablespoon honey
¼ cup bread crumbs
½ cup finely chopped almonds, lightly toasted
½ teaspoon dried thyme
Fine-grained kosher salt and freshly ground black pepper, to taste
4 (4-ounce) salmon steaks

1. Preheat the oven to 350 degrees F.

2. Combine the olive oil with the honey. (Soften the honey in the microwave for 15 seconds, if necessary, for easier blending.)

3. In a shallow dish, combine the bread crumbs, almonds, and thyme, and season with salt and pepper.

4. Coat the salmon with the olive oil mixture and then the almond mixture.

5. Place the salmon on a baking sheet brushed with olive oil and bake 8 to 12 minutes, or until the almonds are lightly browned and the salmon is firm.

Seafood and Poultry Dishes

CALORIES **565**
TOTAL FAT **27 G**
CHOLESTEROL **67 MG**
SATURATED FAT **5 G**
TOTAL CARBOHYDRATES **14 G**

FIBER **1 G**
SUGAR **5 G**
SODIUM **166 MG**
PROTEIN **24 G**

Clam Spaghetti

SERVES 4

PREPARATION TIME **15 MINUTES**
COOKING TIME **15 MINUTES (PLUS TIME TO COOK THE PASTA)**
TOTAL TIME **30 MINUTES (PLUS TIME TO COOK THE PASTA)**

Nothing could be simpler for a weeknight meal than this easy pasta dish.

¼ cup olive oil
1 medium onion, diced
1 medium green bell pepper, cored, seeded, and diced
4 garlic cloves, minced
½ cup chopped fresh flat-leaf parsley, chopped
⅓ teaspoon cayenne pepper
Fine-grained kosher salt and freshly ground black pepper, to taste
3 dozen or so clams, depending on their size
½ cup white wine
1 pound whole-wheat spaghetti
1 lemon, cut into wedges for garnish
½ cup freshly grated, low-fat Parmesan cheese for garnish

1. Heat the olive oil in a large skillet over medium heat. Add the onion, pepper, and garlic, and cook until the onion is translucent. Add the parsley and cayenne pepper, season with salt and pepper, and set aside.

2. Bring a pot of water to a boil. Add the clams and boil for 10 minutes, or until they open (discard any unopened clams). Remove the clams from the pot, reserving the liquid, and shell half of them.

3. Return the skillet to medium-high heat. Add the shelled clams to the skillet, along with the remaining clams, white wine, and 2 cups of the liquid used to boil the clams.

4. Cook the pasta according to the package directions for al dente, drain, and place in a large serving dish.

5. Ladle the clam mixture over the pasta, and toss to serve. Garnish with lemon wedges and Parmesan cheese.

CALORIES **647**
TOTAL FAT **21 G**
CHOLESTEROL **42 MG**
SATURATED FAT **4 G**
TOTAL CARBOHYDRATES **92 G**

FIBER **13 G**
SUGAR **1 G**
SODIUM **660 MG**
PROTEIN **32 G**

Cod Gratin

SERVES 4

PREPARATION TIME **10 MINUTES**
COOKING TIME **20 TO 22 MINUTES**
TOTAL TIME **30 TO 32 MINUTES**

A gratin is any dish with a crispy topping of bread crumbs or cheese. In this tasty French-inspired dish, cod, leeks, and olives peek out from a whole-wheat bread-crumb crust. Serve with sautéed greens, such as spinach, chard, or kale.

½ cup olive oil, divided
1 pound fresh cod
1 cup black kalamata olives, pitted and chopped
4 leeks, trimmed and sliced
1 cup whole-wheat bread crumbs
¾ cup low-sodium chicken stock
Fine-grained kosher salt and freshly ground black pepper, to taste

1. Preheat the oven to 350 degrees F. Brush 4 gratin dishes and a large baking dish with the olive oil.

2. Place the cod in the large baking dish, and bake for 5 to 7 minutes. Cool and cut into 1-inch pieces.

3. Heat the remaining olive oil in a large skillet. Add the olives and leeks, and cook over medium-low heat until the leeks are tender. Add the bread crumbs and chicken stock, stirring to mix. Gently fold in the pieces of cod.

4. Divide the mixture between the 4 gratin dishes, and drizzle with olive oil. Season with salt and pepper.

5. Bake for 15 minutes or until warmed through.

CALORIES **578**
TOTAL FAT **36 G**
CHOLESTEROL **40 MG**
SATURATED FAT **5 G**
TOTAL CARBOHYDRATES **32 G**

FIBER **3 G**
SUGAR **5 G**
SODIUM **623 MG**
PROTEIN **25 G**

Seafood and Poultry Dishes

Halibut with Roasted Vegetables

SERVES 6

PREPARATION TIME **20 MINUTES**
COOKING TIME **25 TO 33 MINUTES**
TOTAL TIME **45 TO 53 MINUTES**

Halibut is a firm, mild fish that pairs well with a variety of seasonings and vegetables. Here, it's combined with tomatoes and zucchini—traditional Mediterranean vegetables—but feel free to improvise with what's available in your garden or at the farmers' market.

¼ cup button mushrooms, coarsely chopped
2 small tomatoes, coarsely chopped
1 small white onion, chopped
2 cups chopped zucchini
2 garlic cloves, minced
1 teaspoon dried herbes de Provence
½ cup olive oil
Fine-grained kosher salt and freshly ground black pepper, to taste
1½ pounds halibut steak, cut into 6 pieces
3 tablespoons finely chopped fresh tarragon
Juice of 1 lemon

1. Preheat the oven to 350 degrees F.

2. Toss the mushrooms, vegetables, and herbs on a large baking sheet with the olive oil, and season with salt and pepper. Roast for 15 to 20 minutes, or until soft and slightly browned. Do not burn.

3. Place the halibut steaks on another baking sheet, and season with the tarragon, salt, pepper, and lemon juice. Roast for 10 to 13 minutes.

4. Top the halibut steaks with the roasted vegetables, and serve.

CALORIES **345**
TOTAL FAT **22 G**
CHOLESTEROL **47 MG**
SATURATED FAT **3 G**
TOTAL CARBOHYDRATES **5 G**

FIBER **1 G**
SUGAR **1 G**
SODIUM **91 MG**
PROTEIN **31 G**

Roasted Sea Bass

SERVES 6

PREPARATION TIME **5 MINUTES**
COOKING TIME **10 TO 15 MINUTES**
TOTAL TIME **15 TO 20 MINUTES**

Roasting is an easy and forgiving way to prepare almost any fish. Use it to cook whole fish, fish fillets, or even fish chunks, and simply adjust the cooking time based on the fish's size. Enjoy this dish with sautéed greens and potatoes.

¼ cup olive oil
6 sea bass filets
Fine-grained kosher salt and freshly ground black pepper, to taste
¼ cup dry white wine
3 teaspoons fresh dill
2 teaspoons fresh thyme
1 garlic clove, minced

1. Preheat the oven to 425 degrees F.

2. Brush the bottom of a roasting pan with olive oil. Place the fish in the pan and brush the fish with oil. Season the fish with salt and pepper. Combine the remaining ingredients and pour them over the fish.

3. Bake for 10 to 15 minutes, depending on the size of the fish. Sea bass is done when the flesh is firm and opaque.

CALORIES **213**
TOTAL FAT **12 G**
CHOLESTEROL **54 MG**
SATURATED FAT **2 G**
TOTAL CARBOHYDRATES **0 G**

FIBER **0 G**
SUGAR **0 G**
SODIUM **88 MG**
PROTEIN **24 G**

Shrimp Salad

SERVES 4

PREPARATION TIME **20 MINUTES (PLUS 3 HOURS TO REFIGERATE)**
COOKING TIME **2 TO 3 MINUTES**
TOTAL TIME **22 MINUTES (PLUS 3 HOURS TO REFIGERATE)**

Main dish salads are a great way to get many servings of vegetables in one meal.
If you prefer to cut down on the sodium content of this dish, use low-salt olives.

2 tablespoons red wine vinegar
Juice of 2 lemons, divided
1 small shallot, finely minced
1 tablespoon chopped fresh mint
¼ teaspoon dried oregano
¼ cup olive oil
Fine-grained kosher salt and freshly ground black pepper, to taste
1 pound shrimp, deveined and shelled
Zest of 1 lemon
1 garlic clove, minced
2 cups baby spinach leaves
1 cup chopped romaine lettuce
½ cup grape tomatoes
1 medium cucumber, peeled, seeded, and diced
½ cup olives, pitted
¼ cup low-fat feta cheese

1. Combine the wine vinegar, half the lemon juice, shallot, chopped mint, and oregano in a bowl. Add the olive oil, whisking constantly for up to 1 minute, or until you create a smooth emulsion. Season with salt and pepper. Refrigerate for 1 hour, and whisk before serving, if it separated.

2. Combine the shrimp with the remaining lemon juice, lemon zest, and garlic in a shallow bowl or bag. Marinate for at least 2 hours.

3. Grill the shrimp in a grill basket or sauté in a frying pan 2 to 3 minutes, or until pink.

4. In a large bowl, toss the greens, tomatoes, cucumber, olives, and feta cheese together. Toss the shrimp with the salad mixture, and drizzle with the vinaigrette. Serve immediately.

CALORIES **213**

TOTAL FAT **20 G**

CHOLESTEROL **177 MG**

SATURATED FAT **4 G**

TOTAL CARBOHYDRATES **8 G**

FIBER **1 G**

SUGAR **1 G**

SODIUM **688 MG**

PROTEIN **27 G**

Meat Dishes

Meat Dishes

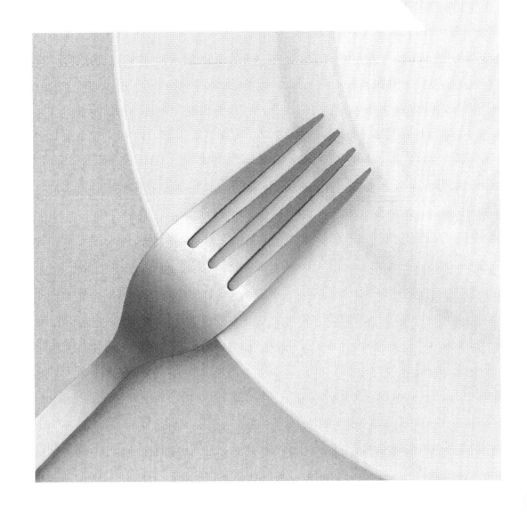

Beef Vegetable Curry

SERVES 6

PREPARATION TIME **15 MINUTES**
COOKING TIME **2 HOURS 15 MINUTES**
TOTAL TIME **2 HOURS 30 MINUTES**

Many people avoid curries because they think the spices will be very hot, but you can avoid the heat very easily by using mild curry. This recipe calls for curry paste rather than powder because the flavor tends to have more depth and complexity, but you can substitute powder if you have it on hand. If mild curry still has a little too much kick for your palate, try serving this dish with cucumber sticks to cool your mouth.

1½ pounds stewing beef, trimmed and cut into ½-inch cubes
1 teaspoon olive oil
1 large onion, chopped
1 large red bell pepper, cored, seeded, and chopped
20 ounces canned diced tomatoes, undrained
1 to 2 tablespoons mild curry paste
1 teaspoon ground cumin
½ teaspoon ground coriander
½ teaspoon fine-grained kosher salt
2 cups green beans, cut into 1-inch pieces
4 cups cooked rice

1. In a large saucepan, brown the beef in the olive oil over medium-high heat, and then transfer the meat to a plate with a slotted spoon. Add the onion and pepper to the saucepan, and sauté until softened. Add the meat back to the saucepan with the diced tomatoes, spices, and salt.

2. Bring the curry to a boil, and then reduce the heat to low. Cover the saucepan and simmer the curry for about 2 hours, or until the meat is very tender.

3. Add the green beans and simmer 5 more minutes.

4. Divide the rice onto 6 plates and top with the beef and vegetable curry to serve.

CALORIES **494**
TOTAL FAT **9 G**
CHOLESTEROL **101 MG**
SATURATED FAT **3 G**
TOTAL CARBOHYDRATES **60 G**

FIBER **5 G**
SUGAR **6 G**
SODIUM **278 MG**
PROTEIN **41 G**

Greek Steak Wraps

SERVES 6

PREPARATION TIME **15 MINUTES**
COOKING TIME **10 MINUTES (PLUS 4 HOURS FOR MARINATING)**
TOTAL TIME **25 MINUTES (PLUS 4 HOURS FOR MARINATING)**

This recipe obviously features lean beef, but it also has other very beneficial elements. One important element is actually one of the most humble: lettuce. Many people think lettuce is just a filler, but it can actually help lower blood pressure, lower bad cholesterol, and cut the risk of inflammation, which are all risk factors associated with diabetes.

¼ cup balsamic vinegar
2 tablespoons olive oil
1 tablespoon minced garlic
1 tablespoon dried oregano
1 tablespoon dried basil
Lemon zest and juice from 1 lemon
Freshly ground black pepper, to taste
1 (18-ounce) flank steak, trimmed completely of fat
6 whole-wheat tortillas
2 cups shredded lettuce
1 medium red onion, sliced thinly
2 cups halved cherry tomatoes

1. Combine the balsamic vinegar, olive oil, garlic, oregano, basil, and lemon zest and juice, and season with pepper. Pour the mixture into a large, resealable plastic bag.

2. Add the steak to the marinade in the bag, turning the bag to coat. Place the sealed bag in the refrigerator on a plate for at least 4 hours or overnight. Turn the bag over several times so that the steak marinates evenly.

3. Preheat a barbecue grill to medium-high heat.

4. Take the steak out of the bag and discard the marinade. Grill the steak 5 minutes per side, or until it is the desired doneness. Remove the steak from the heat and let it rest for at least 10 minutes.

5. Slice the steak diagonally into thin strips.

6. Fill the 6 tortillas with sliced steak, lettuce, onion, and cherry tomatoes, and serve.

CALORIES **347**

TOTAL FAT **13 G**

CHOLESTEROL **47 MG**

SATURATED FAT **4 G**

TOTAL CARBOHYDRATES **28 G**

FIBER **5 G**

SUGAR **1 G**

SODIUM **186 MG**

PROTEIN **28 G**

Meat Dishes

Braised Pork Chops with Spiced Apples

SERVES 4

PREPARATION TIME **30 MINUTES**
COOKING TIME **1 HOUR 20 MINUTES**
TOTAL TIME **1 HOUR 50 MINUTES**

This recipe is a healthier version of a traditional German dish featuring apples and pork. Instead of spoons of butter, wine, and sugar, the sauce in this dish is made with apples and the tang of Dijon mustard. Pectin, which is the soluble fiber in apples, is instrumental for controlling blood sugar because it helps slow the release of blood sugar into the bloodstream.

4 (5-ounce) boneless pork chops, trimmed of fat
1 tablespoon olive oil
1 small onion, thinly sliced
2 large apples, peeled, cored, and cut into thick slices
⅓ cup unsweetened apple juice
1 tablespoon Dijon mustard
¼ teaspoon ground cinnamon
¼ teaspoon ground cumin
1 teaspoon chopped fresh thyme
Pinch of fine-grained kosher salt

1. Preheat the oven to 350 degrees F.

2. Place a large oven-safe skillet over medium-high heat, and brown the pork chops on both sides in olive oil. Remove pork chops from the skillet and set aside on a plate.

3. Add the onion to the skillet and sauté until softened. When the onion is soft add the apples and sauté until the apples are softened. Add the apple juice, mustard, cinnamon, cumin, and thyme to the skillet.

4. Use a slotted spoon to push the apples and onion over to one side of the skillet. Transfer the pork chops and any accumulated juices back into the skillet in one layer.

5. Spoon the apples and onion over the pork chops, and cover the skillet with a lid or foil.

6. Place the skillet in the preheated oven, and bake the pork chops until they are cooked through and very tender, about 1 hour.

7. Season lightly with salt, and serve.

CALORIES **240**

TOTAL FAT **6G**

CHOLESTEROL **80 MG**

SATURATED FAT **2 G**

TOTAL CARBOHYDRATES **21 G**

FIBER **3 G**

SUGAR **11 G**

SODIUM **86 MG**

PROTEIN **26 G**

Meat Dishes

Beef Stroganoff

SERVES 6

PREPARATION TIME **25 MINUTES**
COOKING TIME **35 MINUTES**
TOTAL TIME **1 HOUR**

If you like tender strips of beef combined with a rich mushroom sherry sauce, this recipe is a great choice. The vibrant green parsley accent is absolutely gorgeous, and studies have shown that this herb can help improve blood sugar levels, which could be valuable for helping with diabetes. If you wish to make this dish ahead or in a double batch, it can be frozen with great results if you leave the yogurt out until you serve it.

¾ pound top sirloin, trimmed and cut into thin strips
1 teaspoon olive oil
1½ cups sliced white mushrooms
1 small onion, finely chopped
1 teaspoon minced fresh garlic
1 tablespoon all-purpose flour
¾ cup fat-free low-sodium beef stock
2 tablespoons sherry
6 tablespoons nonfat yogurt
4 teaspoons chopped parsley
Freshly ground black pepper, to taste

1. Place a large skillet over medium-high heat, and sauté the sirloin strips in the oil until browned. Remove the beef from the pan with a slotted spoon, and set aside on a plate.

2. Add the mushrooms, onion, and garlic to the skillet, and sauté them until they are lightly caramelized.

3. Stir in the flour until the vegetables are evenly coated, and then whisk in beef stock and sherry until smooth.

4. Add the browned beef back to the skillet along with any accumulated juices, and stir to combine. Heat over medium heat until the sauce has thickened, stirring constantly.

5. Reduce heat to low and continue to cook until the beef is very tender and the sauce is glossy, about 35 minutes.

6. Stir in the yogurt, top with the parsley, season with pepper, and serve.

CALORIES **167**

TOTAL FAT **5 G**

CHOLESTEROL **52 MG**

SATURATED FAT **2 G**

TOTAL CARBOHYDRATES **7 G**

FIBER **0 G**

SUGAR **1 G**

SODIUM **129 MG**

PROTEIN **19 G**

Grilled Steaks with Sweet Pepper Salsa

SERVES 8

PREPARATION TIME **15 MINUTES (PLUS 1 HOUR MINIMUM FOR MARINATING)**
COOKING TIME **30 MINUTES**
TOTAL TIME **45 MINUTES (PLUS 1 HOUR MINIMUM FOR MARINATING)**

Sometimes simple is best when it comes to sauces or toppings for steaks. The grilled pepper salsa featured in this dish is very simple to make and looks stunning on the plate.

Some people dislike leaving the skin on the bell peppers, so you can remove it before chopping if you allow an extra 10 minutes before grilling the steaks. Simply remove the hot grilled peppers from the barbecue, and place them in a stainless steel bowl and cover it tightly with plastic wrap. Let the peppers steam for about 10 minutes, and peel the loosened skin right off.

4 (10-ounce) beef steaks, trimmed and chopped 1 inch thick
1 tablespoon and 2 teaspoons olive oil, divided
1 tablespoon garlic powder
1 teaspoon ground paprika
2 teaspoons dried oregano
1 teaspoon dried thyme
1 teaspoon freshly ground black pepper
½ teaspoon cayenne pepper
2 red bell peppers, cored, seeded, and cut into quarters
1 yellow bell pepper, cored, seeded, and cut into quarters
1 orange bell pepper, cored, seeded, and cut into quarters
2 tablespoons balsamic vinegar
2 teaspoons chopped fresh basil

1. Brush the steaks with 2 teaspoons of the olive oil, and set aside.

2. In a small bowl stir together the garlic powder, paprika, oregano, thyme, pepper, and cayenne.

3. Rub the spice and herb mixture all over the meat. Cover the steaks, and chill them for at least 1 hour.

4. Preheat grill to medium-high heat.

5. Toss the peppers in a small bowl with the rest of the olive oil and the balsamic vinegar to coat. Grill the peppers until softened and lightly charred, turning.

6. Remove them from the grill and chop them coarsely. Transfer them to a bowl and add the basil; stir to combine, then set aside.

7. Place the steaks on the barbecue, and grill until desired doneness, turning once, about 12 to 15 minutes total for medium rare.

8. Cut the steaks in half, and serve with the grilled peppers.

CALORIES **355**

TOTAL FAT **24 G**

CHOLESTEROL **95 MG**

SATURATED FAT **9 G**

TOTAL CARBOHYDRATES **6 G**

FIBER **1 G**

SUGAR **2 G**

SODIUM **249 MG**

PROTEIN **28 G**

Meat Dishes

Sesame Beef Stir-Fry

SERVES 4

PREPARATION TIME **30 MINUTES**
COOKING TIME **15 MINUTES**
TOTAL TIME **45 MINUTES**

Stir-fry is a cooking technique that can be used in any season and weather because the finished dish is hot but not overly heavy, thanks to all the fresh vegetables and lean meats. Sesame oil and toasted sesame seeds provide a delicious nutty flavor to this dish along with a satisfying crunch. Though they're tiny, sesame seeds pack a great deal of minerals and nutrients along with amino acids and calcium. To get the best flavor, make sure you toast them by tossing them dry in a skillet over medium heat until lightly browned.

½ cup fresh orange juice

3 teaspoons low-sodium tamari or soy sauce

1 tablespoon grated fresh gingerroot

2 teaspoons toasted sesame oil

1 teaspoon cornstarch

Zest from ½ orange

1 teaspoon olive oil

8 ounces boneless beef sirloin, thinly sliced on a bias

2 garlic cloves, minced

½ cup bias-sliced green onions

1 cup snow peas, strings removed and cut in half

1 cup bean sprouts

2 oranges, peeled and sectioned

2 teaspoons toasted sesame seeds

2 cups hot, cooked brown rice

1. In a small bowl whisk together the orange juice, tamari, gingerroot, sesame oil, cornstarch, and orange zest; set aside.

2. Place a large skillet over medium-high heat and add the olive oil. Stir-fry the beef for 4 minutes until desired doneness. Add the garlic, green onions, snow peas, and bean sprouts, and stir-fry for about 4 minutes.

3. Move the meat and vegetables to the side of the pan and add the sauce. Stir until the sauce has thickened and is bubbly. Stir the meat and vegetables into the sauce to coat.

4. Add the orange segments and toasted sesame seeds. Serve over hot, cooked brown rice (½ cup per serving).

CALORIES **410**

TOTAL FAT **11 G**

CHOLESTEROL **76 MG**

SATURATED FAT **3 G**

TOTAL CARBOHYDRATES **44 G**

FIBER **5 G**

SUGAR **14 G**

SODIUM **587 MG**

PROTEIN **34 G**

Stuffed Peppers

SERVES 8

PREPARATION TIME **15 MINUTES**
COOKING TIME **35 MINUTES**
TOTAL TIME **50 MINUTES**

Comfort food has never been healthier than this version of stuffed peppers. You can easily double or even triple this recipe with little effort if you have a great horde of people to feed. Peppers are the perfect sweet container to hold the savory filling. All colors of peppers contain lots of vitamin A and C along with many vitamins, folic acid, potassium, and niacin. Try using an assortment of shades to create an interesting display of stuffed peppers.

4 large red or yellow bell peppers, cored, cut in half lengthwise, and seeded
1 pound extra-lean ground beef
1 stalk celery, diced
1 small onion, finely chopped
1 teaspoon minced garlic
1 cup cooked brown rice
2 small tomatoes, chopped
½ cup frozen and thawed or fresh corn
1 teaspoon dried basil
¼ teaspoon fine-grained kosher salt
¼ teaspoon freshly ground black pepper
½ cup water

1. Preheat the oven to 350 degrees F.

2. Place the peppers in a 13 × 9–inch baking pan, skin-side down.

3. In a large skillet placed over medium-high heat, cook the ground beef, celery, and onion until the beef is cooked through and the onion is soft. Add the garlic and sauté another minute.

4. Remove from the heat and drain off the fat. Stir the cooked rice, tomatoes, corn, basil, salt, and pepper into the beef mixture in skillet. Spoon the mixture into pepper halves.

5. Pour water around the stuffed peppers, and cover the baking dish with foil. Bake the peppers for about 30 minutes; then uncover and bake an additional 5 minutes.

CALORIES **396**

TOTAL FAT **7 G**

CHOLESTEROL **60 MG**

SATURATED FAT **2 G**

TOTAL CARBOHYDRATES **54 G**

FIBER **7 G**

SUGAR **10 G**

SODIUM **232 MG**

PROTEIN **30 G**

Meat Dishes

Slow Cooker Italian-Style Pork Chops

SERVES 6

PREPARATION TIME **15 MINUTES**
COOKING TIME **8 TO 9 HOURS ON LOW OR 4 TO 5 HOURS ON HIGH**
TOTAL TIME **VARIES DEPENDING ON HEAT SETTING**

Creating simple tasty meals in a slow cooker is incredibly convenient and lovely to come home to after a long day at work or school. You can add other vegetables to this recipe depending on what is in your crisper, such as celery, eggplant, mushrooms, or carrots. They will add flavor to the stock and be delightful combined with the tender pork and hearty tomato sauce.

1 large onion, coarsely chopped
6 pork chops (bone in), trimmed
1 teaspoon dried basil
1 teaspoon dried oregano
4 teaspoons minced garlic
½ teaspoon fine-grained kosher salt
½ teaspoon freshly ground black pepper
6 large tomatoes, chopped, with accumulated juices
4 teaspoons balsamic vinegar
2 medium zucchini, diced
4 teaspoons cornstarch
4 teaspoons cold water

1. Place half the onion in a slow cooker. Place three of the pork chops over the onion. Sprinkle them with half the basil, oregano, garlic, salt, and pepper. Repeat these layers with the remaining onion, pork chops, herbs, garlic, salt, and pepper. Top the layers with the tomatoes, balsamic vinegar, and zucchini.

2. Cover and cook on low heat for 8 to 9 hours or on high heat for 4 to 5 hours.

3. Use a slotted spoon to transfer the pork chops and vegetables to a serving plate and cover to keep warm.

4. Pour the cooking juices from the slow cooker into a medium saucepan, and place it over medium-high heat.

5. Whisk together the cornstarch and water in a small bowl, and add it to the cooking juices. Cook until the sauce is thick and bubbling.

6. Serve the sauce over the pork chops and vegetables.

CALORIES **333**

TOTAL FAT **20 G**

CHOLESTEROL **69 MG**

SATURATED FAT **8 G**

TOTAL CARBOHYDRATES **17 G**

FIBER **4 G**

SUGAR **8 G**

SODIUM **228 MG**

PROTEIN **21 G**

Slow Cooker Venison Roast

SERVES 10

PREPARATION TIME **5 MINUTES**
COOKING TIME **10 HOURS**
TOTAL TIME **10 HOURS 5 MINUTES**

Venison is a very healthful meat choice because it is low in fat and cholesterol. Deer are not factory-farmed, which means venison is not full of hormones and antibiotics. You can season this roast with any combination of herbs to create the right flavor for the meat.

2 pounds venison roast, trimmed
2 tablespoons cider vinegar
1 tablespoon maple syrup
1 teaspoon ground cinnamon
½ teaspoon fine-grained kosher salt
½ teaspoon freshly ground black pepper

1. Place the roast in a slow cooker, and add enough water just to cover it.

2. Add the vinegar, maple syrup, cinnamon, salt, and pepper, and stir to mix into the water.

3. Set the slow cooker on high, and when the liquid starts to boil, after about 2 hours, reduce the temperature to low and cook for about 8 hours until the meat is tender.

4. Remove the venison from the slow cooker and serve.

CALORIES **138**
TOTAL FAT **2 G**
CHOLESTEROL **77 MG**
SATURATED FAT **1 G**
TOTAL CARBOHYDRATES **2 G**

FIBER **0 G**
SUGAR **1 G**
SODIUM **41 MG**
PROTEIN **29 G**

Indonesian Pork Tenderloin

SERVES 4

PREPARATION TIME **10 MINUTES (PLUS 3 HOURS MINIMUM FOR MARINATING)**
COOKING TIME **15 TO 20 MINUTES**
TOTAL TIME **25 TO 30 MINUTES (PLUS 3 HOURS MINIMUM FOR MARINATING)**

The marinade used for this fragrant pork tenderloin can also be paired with chicken with lovely results. It is very important to use fresh gingerroot in this dish so that the flavor is strong enough and you get all the wonderful health benefits associated with ginger. Ginger is an anti-inflammatory and is thought to help treat many ailments, such as migraines, heartburn, and high blood pressure.

¼ cup fresh lime juice
1 teaspoon lime zest
1 tablespoon low-sodium soy sauce
5 teaspoons grated fresh gingerroot
1 teaspoon crushed red pepper flakes
4 teaspoons minced garlic
1½ pounds pork tenderloin, trimmed of fat

1. In a medium bowl, whisk together everything except the pork tenderloin, and pour half the marinade into a large, resealable plastic bag. (Reserve the other half of the marinade in a bowl in the refrigerator.) Add the pork to the bag and seal it, turning a few times to coat the meat. Store the bag in the refrigerator at least 3 hours or overnight.

2. Preheat the barbecue grill to medium-high heat, and take the pork out of the refrigerator.

3. Drain the pork and grill for about 15 minutes, turning and basting with the reserved marinade until the internal temperature reads 160 degrees F. Serve warm.

CALORIES **263**
TOTAL FAT **6 G**
CHOLESTEROL **124 MG**
SATURATED FAT **2 G**
TOTAL CARBOHYDRATES **5 G**

FIBER **1G**
SUGAR **1 G**
SODIUM **249 MG**
PROTEIN **45 G**

Desserts

Coconut Pie

Strawberry Shortcake

Orange Panna Cotta

Sugar Cookies

Rich Chocolate Torte

Apple Tart

Coffee Custards

Vanilla Rice Pudding

Dark Chocolate Sherbet

Traditional Pear Crisp

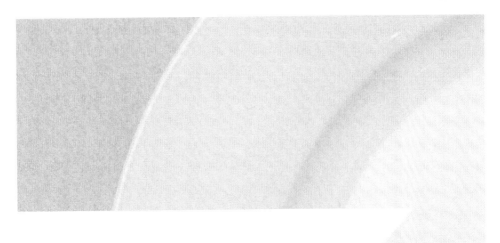

CHAPTER THIRTEEN
Desserts

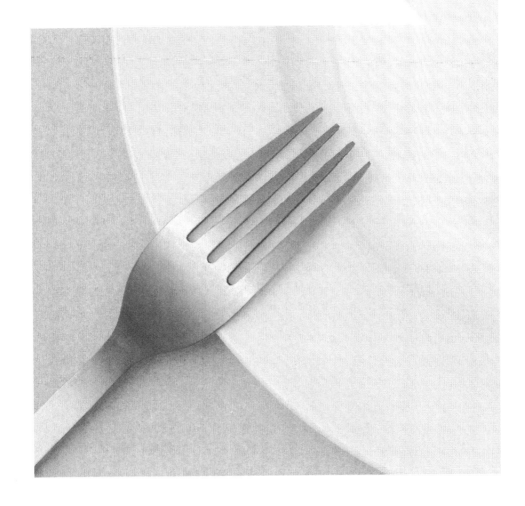

Coconut Pie

SERVES 8

PREPARATION TIME **15 MINUTES**
COOKING TIME **30 MINUTES**
TOTAL TIME **45 MINUTES**

This pie has a very nice coconut taste that can be enhanced further with the addition of coconut extract in the filling. Coconut is a very nutrient-dense fruit, which can be very effective for improving the digestion and boosting energy. If you use packaged coconut rather than fresh, make sure you buy the unsweetened variety to reduce the sugar in the final dish. You can use your own favorite pie crust recipe if you don't want the convenience of premade products.

4 large eggs, at room temperature
2 cups nonfat milk
Sugar-free sweetener equivalent to 1 cup granulated sugar
4 teaspoons cornstarch
½ teaspoon salt
¾ cup flaked unsweetened coconut, toasted
1 single-crust 9-inch pie shell, premade

1. Preheat the oven to 375 degrees F.

2. In a large bowl, beat the eggs with a hand beater for about 5 minutes, or until very thick and pale-lemon colored.

3. Whisk in the milk, sweetener, cornstarch, salt, and coconut until well combined.

4. Pour the coconut mixture into the pie shell.

5. Bake the pie for 30 minutes, or until a sharp knife inserted in the center comes out clean.

6. Cool the pie on a wire rack.

7. Serve at room temperature or chilled.

CALORIES **169**
TOTAL FAT **10 G**
CHOLESTEROL **94 MG**
SATURATED FAT **4 G**
TOTAL CARBOHYDRATES **13 G**

FIBER **1 G**
SUGAR **5 G**
SODIUM **312 MG**
PROTEIN **6 G**

Strawberry Shortcake

SERVES 6

PREPARATION TIME **20 MINUTES**
COOKING TIME **10 MINUTES**
TOTAL TIME **30 MINUTES**

Modern shortcake recipes often call for a pound cake base, but traditional variations, like this one, actually use a sweetened biscuit. This recipe could easily be switched to include any kind of berry, stone fruit such as peaches, plums, or nectarines, and even lovely apples or pears. Try to make the original version with ripe, plump strawberries at least once to see how gorgeous the golden biscuit, creamy white yogurt, and vibrant red berries look together on the plate. Very festive!

2 cups whole-wheat pastry flour, sifted
¼ cup all-purpose flour, sifted
3 teaspoons low-sodium baking powder
2 teaspoons sweetener
¼ cup chilled almond butter
¾ cup nonfat milk
1 cup plain nonfat yogurt
6 cups fresh strawberries, washed, hulled, and sliced

1. Preheat the oven to 350 degrees F, and line a baking sheet with parchment paper; set aside.

2. In a large bowl, sift together the whole-wheat flour, all-purpose flour, baking powder, and sweetener.

3. Add the chilled almond butter, and use a fork to cut it into the dry ingredients until the mixture resembles coarse meal.

4. Add the milk and toss together just until a moist dough forms.

5. Transfer the dough to a floured cutting board or counter, and knead it gently with floured hands until it holds together well and is smooth.

6. Roll out the dough into a ¼-inch-thick rectangle, and cut out 12 round shortcakes. You might have to gather up the scraps and reroll the dough if needed.

7. Transfer the shortcakes onto the baking sheet, and bake 8 to 10 minutes, or until golden.

8. Let the shortcakes cool and then place one on each plate. Top each shortcake with yogurt and fresh berries. Then top the berries with a second shortcake. Enjoy!

CALORIES **335**

FIBER **4 G**

TOTAL FAT **7 G**

SUGAR **14 G**

CHOLESTEROL **3 MG**

SODIUM **202 MG**

SATURATED FAT **1 G**

PROTEIN **11 G**

TOTAL CARBOHYDRATES **56 G**

Orange Panna Cotta

SERVES 6

PREPARATION TIME **20 MINUTES**
COOKING TIME **10 MINUTES (PLUS 6 HOURS MINIMUM FOR CHILLING)**
TOTAL TIME **30 MINUTES (PLUS 6 HOURS MINIMUM FOR CHILLING)**

Panna cotta is a dessert that is incredibly simple to make and has its roots in Italy. It has a pleasing delicate texture that melts on the tongue and leaves you feeling refreshed rather than overly full. Make sure you chill it for the recommended time so that the panna cotta sets perfectly.

3 tablespoons sweetener
1 tablespoon unflavored gelatin powder
1⅓ cup nonfat milk
1¼ cup Greek yogurt
1 teaspoon almond extract, divided
1 teaspoon cornstarch
½ cup fresh orange juice (no sugar added)
1 can tangerine segments, packed in juice and drained

1. In a small pan, whisk together the sweetener and gelatin powder.

2. Put the pan over medium-low heat and whisk in the milk, stirring constantly until the sugar and gelatin are dissolved. Remove from the heat.

3. Whisk in the yogurt and half the almond extract until the mixture is very smooth.

4. Pour the panna cotta mixture into the ramekins, dividing evenly.

5. Cover and chill the panna cotta for at least 6 hours or until set.

6. Whisk together the cornstarch and orange juice in a small saucepan, and heat over medium-high heat until the mixture has thickened.

7. Remove from the heat, and stir in the remaining almond extract and tangerine segments. Cool completely in the refrigerator.

8. To serve, dip the bottom halves of the ramekins in hot water for about 10 seconds, and then run a sharp knife around the edges to loosen the panna cotta. Invert serving plates over each of the ramekins and then turn the plate and ramekin over together. Remove the ramekin and top the panna cotta with sauce.

CALORIES **106**

TOTAL FAT **1 G**

CHOLESTEROL **4 MG**

SATURATED FAT **0 G**

TOTAL CARBOHYDRATES **19 G**

FIBER **1 G**

SUGAR **16 G**

SODIUM **55 MG**

PROTEIN **6 G**

Sugar Cookies

SERVES 24

PREPARATION TIME **15 MINUTES (PLUS 1 HOUR FOR CHILLING)**
COOKING TIME **10 TO 12 MINUTES**
TOTAL TIME **25 TO 27 MINUTES (PLUS 1 HOUR FOR CHILLING)**

These cookies are a perfect light dessert and can be served plain with a fragrant rich cup of coffee or jazzed up with fresh fruit for a real treat. The dominant taste in these tender morsels is vanilla. This popular flavoring has many health benefits if you use real vanilla extract or the entire bean. The B-complex vitamins in vanilla can help regulate and stabilize the metabolism, which is important for anyone with diabetes.

¾ cup mashed avocado
¼ cup butter
Sugar-free equivalent of ½ cup granulated sugar
1 tablespoon pure vanilla extract
2 large egg whites
4 tablespoons water
¼ teaspoon white vinegar
1¾ cups whole-wheat flour, sifted
½ cup cake flour, sifted
1 teaspoon baking powder
⅛ teaspoon salt

1. Preheat the oven to 350 degrees F. Line a cookie sheet with parchment paper; set aside.

2. In a large bowl, beat together the avocado, butter, sweetener, and vanilla until very well blended.

3. Beat in the egg whites, water, and vinegar, scraping down the sides of the bowl a few times. Set aside.

4. In a medium bowl, combine the whole-wheat flour, cake flour, baking powder, and salt. Add the dry ingredients to the wet ingredients, and mix together until a sticky dough forms.

5. Divide the dough into two balls, and wrap them in plastic wrap. Place the dough balls in the refrigerator for at least 1 hour or until the dough is firm enough to roll out.

6. Generously flour a flat work surface, and roll out the dough balls until each is ¼ inch thick.

7. Cut the cookies out with your favorite cookie cutters, and place them on the prepared tray. You might have to gather up the dough scraps and roll the dough out again.

8. Bake cookies for about 10 to 12 minutes, or until they are very lightly browned on the bottoms.

9. Cool cookies on a wire rack.

CALORIES **70**

TOTAL FAT **3 G**

CHOLESTEROL **5 MG**

SATURATED FAT **1 G**

TOTAL CARBOHYDRATES **10 G**

FIBER **1 G**

SUGAR **4 G**

SODIUM **31 MG**

PROTEIN **2 G**

Desserts

Rich Chocolate Torte

SERVES 16

PREPARATION TIME **30 MINUTES**
COOKING TIME **20 TO 25 MINUTES**
TOTAL TIME **50 TO 55 MINUTES**

Nothing beats the dense rich goodness of a terrific chocolate cake after a good meal. This dark beauty uses unsweetened chocolate and coffee to create an unforgettable flavor. Chocolate is widely accepted as a healthful addition to any diet because it is packed full of antioxidants, which can help regulate blood sugar and support a healthy cardiovascular system.

8 tablespoons butter or margarine, plus more to grease the pan
5 ounces unsweetened chocolate, chopped
½ cup nonfat milk
¼ cup sugar-free apricot jam
3 teaspoons instant coffee granules
2 large egg yolks
1 tablespoon pure vanilla extract
Sugar-free sweetener equivalent to 1½ cups granulated sugar
4 egg whites, at room temperature
¼ teaspoon cream of tartar
⅓ cup all-purpose flour
⅛ teaspoon salt
1 cup fresh raspberries

1. Preheat the oven to 350 degrees F, and lightly grease an 8-inch springform pan with butter. Line the pan with parchment paper, and lightly grease the parchment; set aside.

2. Place the 8 tablespoons of butter, chocolate, milk, apricot jam, and coffee in a small saucepan over low heat, and whisk until the chocolate is melted and the mixture is smooth.

3. Remove the saucepan from the heat, and whisk in the egg yolks, vanilla, and sweetener until smooth. Cool completely.

4. In a large bowl, beat the egg whites and cream of tartar until stiff peaks form. Fold in the cooled chocolate mixture, and then fold in the flour and salt. Try to keep as much volume in the batter as possible.

5. Spoon cake batter into the prepared pan, and smooth down the top with a spatula. Bake the cake in the center of the preheated oven for 20 to 25 minutes, or until a toothpick inserted in the center comes out clean.

6. Remove the cake from the oven, and run a sharp knife around the edges of the pan to loosen the cake from the pan.

7. Place the cake on a wire rack, and cool completely. Cover the pan and place the cake in the refrigerator for 1 to 2 hours or until completely chilled.

8. Remove the cake from the springform pan, and garnish with fresh raspberries.

CALORIES **143**

TOTAL FAT **11 G**

CHOLESTEROL **26 MG**

SATURATED FAT **4 G**

TOTAL CARBOHYDRATES **11 G**

FIBER **2 G**

SUGAR **1 G**

SODIUM **107 MG**

PROTEIN **3 G**

Apple Tart

SERVES 12

PREPARATION TIME **30 MINUTES (PLUS 1 HOUR FOR CHILLING
    THE DOUGH)**
COOKING TIME **50 TO 55 MINUTES**
TOTAL TIME **1 HOUR 20 MINUTES TO 1 HOUR 25 MINUTES (PLUS
    1 HOUR FOR CHILLING THE DOUGH)**

*The tart shell in this recipe could become a new staple recipe for all your other
flan and tart creations because it is delicious and a healthier alternative.
Some people think that oats need to be avoided when you have diabetes, but
this is actually not the case. Oats contain a variety of nutrients and minerals
and are very easy to digest. They are a superfood, which assists in controlling
blood pressure, cholesterol, and blood sugar levels.*

1 cup quick-cooking rolled oats
½ cup whole-wheat flour
¼ cup ground pecans
1 cup nonfat cream cheese, softened, divided
3 teaspoons butter, softened
3 teaspoons sweetener
¼ teaspoon baking soda
Pinch of salt
¼ cup nonfat sour cream
1 large egg white
6 teaspoons sugar-free orange marmalade, divided
¼ teaspoon ground nutmeg
3 medium tart red apples, peeled, cored, and very thinly sliced

1. In a medium bowl, stir together the oats, whole-wheat flour, and pecans
until well mixed; set aside.

2. In another medium bowl, beat together ½ cup of cream cheese and the
butter until well combined.

3. Add the sweetener, baking soda, and salt, and beat until mixed thoroughly.
Stir in the oat mixture until mixed in.

4. Gather the dough into a ball, cover, and place it in the refrigerator until it is well chilled (30 to 60 minutes).

5. Preheat the oven to 375 degrees F, and lightly grease a 9-inch tart pan.

6. Pat the dough into the bottom and sides of the tart pan. Line the pastry with lightly oiled foil, and bake for about 5 minutes.

7. Remove the foil and bake the shell for about 5 minutes more. Cool the tart shell for about 15 minutes on a wire rack.

8. Meanwhile, make the filling. In a medium bowl, blend the remaining cream cheese, sour cream, egg white, 3 teaspoons of the orange marmalade, and nutmeg until very smooth.

9. Spread the cream cheese filling into the cooled crust. Arrange the apple slices in a pretty pattern on top of the cream cheese filling, and cover the top of the tart with foil.

10. Bake the tart for 30 to 35 minutes, and then uncover it and bake 10 minutes more, or until the crust is golden.

11. Melt the remaining orange marmalade in the microwave on 50 percent power. Brush the melted marmalade over the apples and serve the tart slightly warm.

CALORIES **121**

TOTAL FAT **3 G**

CHOLESTEROL **6 MG**

SATURATED FAT **1 G**

TOTAL CARBOHYDRATES **18 G**

FIBER **3 G**

SUGAR **7 G**

SODIUM **191 MG**

PROTEIN **6 G**

Coffee Custards

SERVES 6

PREPARATION TIME **20 MINUTES**
COOKING TIME **30 TO 40 MINUTES**
TOTAL TIME **50 MINUTES TO 1 HOUR (PLUS 4 TO 6 HOURS FOR CHILLING)**

Custards are a lovely choice for dessert on warm summer and fall evenings because they are so cool and creamy. Coffee adds a certain sophistication to this unpretentious dessert, which can be played up by garnishing each custard with a chocolate-dipped coffee bean.

2¼ cups nonfat milk
Sugar-free sweetener equivalent to ¼ cup granulated sugar
¼ cup cocoa powder
2 teaspoons instant coffee granules
1 cup eggs, about 4 large beaten
1 tablespoon pure vanilla extract

1. Preheat the oven to 325 degrees F. Place six 6-ounce ramekins in a large rectangular baking dish.

2. In a saucepan, whisk together the milk, sweetener, cocoa powder, and coffee.

3. Place the pan over medium heat, and cook, stirring until the cocoa and coffee are dissolved.

4. Place the eggs in a medium bowl, and whisk the hot mixture into them slowly. Whisk in the vanilla.

5. Pour the egg mixture through a fine sieve into a pitcher, and then fill the ramekins, dividing equally.

6. Pour boiling water around the ramekins to a depth of about 1 inch.

7. Bake the custards for 30 to 40 minutes, or until a knife inserted in the center comes out clean.

8. Remove the ramekins from baking dish, and cool to room temperature.

9. Transfer them to the refrigerator and chill until firm (4 to 6 hours).

CALORIES **78**

TOTAL FAT **4 G**

CHOLESTEROL **114 MG**

SATURATED FAT **1 G**

TOTAL CARBOHYDRATES **5 G**

FIBER **1 G**

SUGAR **4 G**

SODIUM **72 MG**

PROTEIN **7 G**

Vanilla Rice Pudding

SERVES 6

PREPARATION TIME **5 MINUTES**
COOKING TIME **45 MINUTES**
TOTAL TIME **50 MINUTES**

Vanilla pudding is not just a satisfying choice for dessert, it is also a great breakfast or snack item as well. This recipe uses a combination of regular nonfat milk and almond milk to create the lovely fragrant sauce. Almond milk is incredibly nutritious and is a wonderful source of vitamin A, vitamin B, vitamin D, and vitamin E. It also contains almost no cholesterol while being low in sodium and calories.

2½ cups nonfat milk
1 cup unsweetened almond milk
1 vanilla bean, split
1½ cup quick-cooking brown rice
1 teaspoon ground cinnamon
¼ teaspoon nutmeg
Pinch of salt
Sugar-free sweetener equivalent to 1 tablespoon sugar, or to taste

1. Place the milk and almond milk in a large saucepan over medium heat. Scrape the seeds from the vanilla bean into the milk, and then add the whole bean as well.

2. Bring the milk mixture to a gentle simmer, and let it simmer for 10 to 15 minutes to infuse the vanilla flavor into the milk.

3. Remove the vanilla bean from the milk, and add the rice, spices, and salt to the saucepan.

4. Cook, stirring frequently until the rice is tender and most of the milk has been absorbed.

5. Stir in the sweetener and serve warm or cold.

CALORIES **213**
TOTAL FAT **2 G**
CHOLESTEROL **2 MG**
SATURATED FAT **0 G**
TOTAL CARBOHYDRATES **43 G**

FIBER **3 G**
SUGAR **5 G**
SODIUM **102 MG**
PROTEIN **7 G**

Dark Chocolate Sherbet

SERVES 12

PREPARATION TIME **5 MINUTES**
COOKING TIME **20 MINUTES (PLUS CHILLING OVERNIGHT AND 2 HOURS FREEZING IN ICE-CREAM MAKER)**
TOTAL TIME **25 MINUTES (PLUS CHILLING OVERNIGHT AND 2 HOURS FREEZING IN ICE-CREAM MAKER)**

This cool rich treat is easy to make if you have an ice cream maker but can also be created with a freezer, a spoon, and a great deal of patience. Simply pour the chilled sherbet mixture into a baking pan and place it in the freezer. Every fifteen to thirty minutes, stir the mixture until it starts to form crystals. Continue to stir and scrape until the sherbet resembles creamy chocolate snow.

8 ounces 75 percent chocolate, chopped
2 cups water
Sugar-free sweetener equivalent to ½ cup granulated sugar
½ cup 2 percent milk
1 tablespoon pure vanilla extract
½ cup hulled and sliced fresh strawberries for garnish

1. In a large saucepan, mix together the chopped chocolate, water, sugar, and milk.

2. Bring the mixture to a boil, whisking constantly.

3. Boil for 1 minute until the chocolate is melted.

4. Remove the saucepan from the heat, and whisk in the vanilla.

5. Transfer the chocolate mixture to a bowl, and chill overnight covered.

6. Freeze the chocolate mixture in an ice-cream maker according to the manufacturer's directions.

7. Scoop the sherbet into dishes and top with strawberries.

CALORIES **133**
TOTAL FAT **16 G**
CHOLESTEROL **1 MG**
SATURATED FAT **6 G**
TOTAL CARBOHYDRATES **9 G**

FIBER **1 G**
SUGAR **7 G**
SODIUM **10 MG**
PROTEIN **3 G**

Traditional Pear Crisp

SERVES 10

PREPARATION TIME **30 MINUTES**
COOKING TIME **45 MINUTES**
TOTAL TIME **1 HOUR 15 MINUTES**

Pear crisp is a nice dessert anytime, but is absolutely perfect for fall and the chilly winds of winter. Pears are a wonderful source of fiber, especially the skins, so leave them on for a healthier dish. The apple butter in the crisp is also packed with insoluble fiber, vitamin A, and vitamin C.

Olive oil cooking spray
¼ cup tapioca starch
½ cup unsweetened apple juice
10 cups cored and sliced pears
4 teaspoons apple butter
2 teaspoons melted butter
1 cup rolled oats
1 teaspoon brown sugar
1 teaspoon ground nutmeg
½ teaspoon ground cinnamon
Pinch of salt

1. Preheat the oven to 325 degrees F, and lightly oil a 9 × 9–inch baking pan with spray; set aside.

2. In a small bowl, whisk together the tapioca and apple juice; set aside for 15 minutes.

3. Add the pear slices to the tapioca mixture, and stir until well combined. Spoon the pears into the greased baking dish.

4. In a large bowl, stir together the apple butter, butter, oats, brown sugar, spices, and salt until the mixture resembles coarse crumbs.

5. Top the pears with the crumble mixture, and cover the baking dish with foil. Bake for 25 minutes covered, and then uncover and bake for an additional 15 to 20 minutes until the top is browned.

6. Serve warm.

CALORIES **160**

TOTAL FAT **2 G**

CHOLESTEROL **2 MG**

SATURATED FAT **1 G**

TOTAL CARBOHYDRATES **37 G**

FIBER **6 G**

SUGAR **19 G**

SODIUM **24 MG**

PROTEIN **2 G**

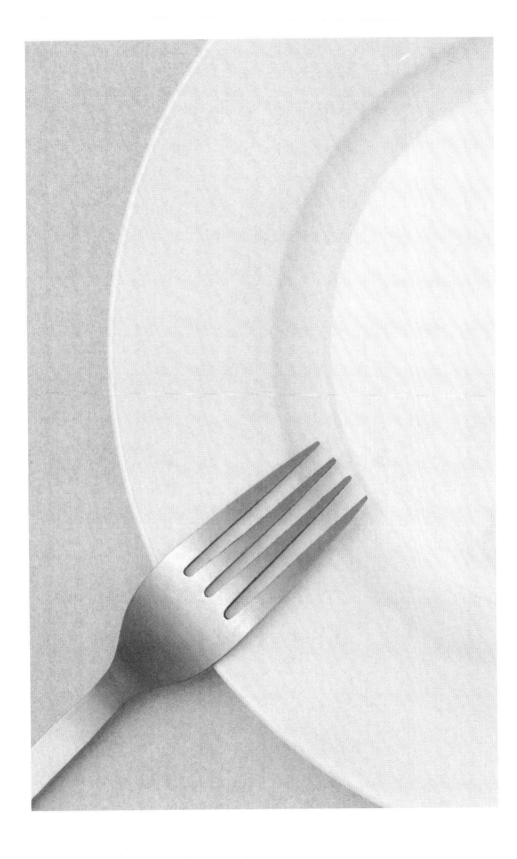

References

American Heart Association. "Coronary Artery Disease—Coronary Heart Disease."
Last modified August 30, 2013. http://www.heart.org/HEARTORG/Conditions/More/
MyHeartandStrokeNews/Coronary-Artery-Disease---Coronary-Heart-Disease_
UCM_436416_Article.jsp

Centers for Disease Control and Prevention. "Alcohol and Public Health: Frequently
Asked Questions." Last modified July 31, 2013. http://www.cdc.gov/alcohol/faqs.htm#6.

National Diabetes Education Program. "The Diabetes Epidemic Among African Americans." Last modified January 2011. http://www.ndep.nih.gov/media/FS_AfricanAm.
pdf?redirect=true.

Appendix: Conversion of Sugar Substitutes

Sweetener	Amount of Sugar	Equivalent Amount of Sweetener
acesulfame potassium	¼ cup	6 grams
agave nectar	1 cup	½ cup
aspartame (Equal, NutraSweet)	¼ cup	6 grams
brown rice malt syrup	1 cup	1 cup
fructose	1 cup	⅔ cup
fruit juice concentrate	1 cup	¾ cup (dry) ¾ cup minus 3 teaspoons (liquid)
honey	1 cup	½ cup
Just Like Sugar (chicory root)	1 cup	1 cup
maple sugar	1 cup	¼ cup
maple syrup	1 cup	½ cup
molasses	1 cup	½ cup
saccharine (Sweet'N Low)	¼ cup	6 grams
stevia	1 cup	⅛ cup
sucralose (Splenda)	1 cup	1 c. (granular)
sucralose-brown sugar blend	1 teaspoon	½ teaspoon
sucralose-sugar blend	1 cup	½ cup
xylitol	1 cup	⅜ cup

Index

253

Index

Index

Index